Topics in Geriatric Care

This book series draws expertise from across the globe to focus on improving the care of older people in hospital, residential aged care, and general practice settings by adopting an evidence-based approach with person-centered care. The different volumes focus on various aspects of the mind, mobility, medications, multimorbidity of older people to meet their expectations. The role of health services, preventive activities, and treatments in maintaining the quality of life for older people are discussed. Many contributors to the series have contributed significantly to the evolution of curriculum, training, and guidelines in the evolving discipline. All the contributors are leaders in their respective fields.

The series editors are internationally renowned geriatricians and gerontologists. This series will change the approach to the practice of geriatrics.

Julie Byles
Editor

What Matters for Healthy Ageing

Springer

BYWORD BOOKS™

Editor
Julie Byles
School of Medicine and Public Health
The University of Newcastle
Newcastle, NSW, Australia

ISSN 2731-5347 ISSN 2731-5355 (electronic)
Topics in Geriatric Care
ISBN 978-981-96-0461-6 ISBN 978-981-96-0462-3 (eBook)
https://doi.org/10.1007/978-981-96-0462-3

Jointly published with Byword Books

This Springer imprint is published by the registered company Springer Nature Singapore Pte Ltd.
The registered company address is: 152 Beach Road, #21-01/04 Gateway East, Singapore 189721, Singapore

Preface

This volume considers healthy ageing from the point of view of the individual. It takes account of both the length of life and the quality life, and all the things that make life worthwhile in later years. These aspects include peoples' roles and identity, participation and activity, capacities, and abilities. The volume embraces the World Health Organization definition of healthy ageing being the maintenance of abilities to be and do the things that bring life value and considering a balance of intrinsic capacity and external support. The volume also considers the social context of ageing, including the effects of socioeconomic status and circumstances across the life course, and the importance of social networks and supports in later life. The works recognize the foundational, cumulative, and life course influences on later life. The works also recognize that later life is a journey full of non-linear transitions. People may continue to work, despite advancing age. Retirement does not mean the end of social participation and contribution, or even the end of work. Disease does not mean disability, and disability does not mean an inability to pursue one's goals. Needing care does not mean one is not contributing to the care of others. At all stages older people retain the capacity to learn, grow, create, and have meaningful relationships. An essential component of healthy ageing is to enable people to participate in life, despite any physical or cognitive difficulties or other limitations.

What matters most to older people themselves has not always been in the domain of policy and practice concerning older populations. Discourse is often centred around structural ageing of the population, dependency ratios, burden of disease, costs of care, care requirements, and other, often negative, constructs of ageing and their effects on society. This approach leads to a pervasive ageism that counts the costs of getting older, without acknowledging the wins. Here we attempt to balance the books, facing the realities of ageing in terms of disease risk and functional decline against the potential for people to make the most of their later years.

Newcastle, NSW, Australia | Julie Byles

Introduction to the Series on "Topics in Geriatric Care"

The population is ageing because of our successful public health measures over the past few decades. Ageing is a global phenomenon. According to the World Health Organization (WHO), 80% of the older people live in middle- to low-income countries. In 2020, the number of people aged 60 years and older outnumbered children younger than 5 years. Moreover, the proportion of the world's population over 60 years will nearly double from 12% to 22%, from 2015 to 2050. Some people describe ageing as a "tsunami", but I differ. Tsunami is unpredictable, but we knew the population was, and is, ageing for several decades. We should have a pro-active, evidence-based approach to ageing and its medical and healthcare needs. With the ageing of the world's population, it has become increasingly important to understand the challenges and opportunities associated with providing high-quality care to older individuals.

WHO has declared the current decade as the decade of Healthy Ageing. So our aim should be to keep the ageing population active, healthy, and happy. In spite of this, ageism is still an issue, both in the wider society and healthcare systems. We know that a majority of older people are independent, in spite of the multimorbidity and chronic diseases. Often an older person is caring for another older person. All healthcare professionals, irrespective of their specialties, should have adequate knowledge in geriatric medicine. Older people suffer from multiple system diseases. Ageing also is risk factor for frailty. This gives us opportunities to intervene in multiple ways.

This series on "Topics in Geriatric Care" is intended to serve as a comprehensive resource for healthcare professionals, researchers, and students around the world who are interested in this field. This series is designed to provide a broad overview of the key topics in geriatric care, with a focus on evidence-based approaches to diagnosis, treatment, and management. It covers a wide range of topics, including the biology of ageing, common geriatric syndromes, psychological issues in ageing, and the social and ethical dimensions of caring for older adults. This series also includes practical information on the assessment and management of common medical conditions in older adults, as well as strategies for promoting healthy ageing and enhancing quality of life. The authors of this series are leading experts in the field of geriatrics, with extensive clinical and research experience with a focus on international best practices and the unique challenges and opportunities associated with providing care to older adults in different parts of the world. Each volume is based on the geriatric syndromes, including what matters to older people, multimorbidity, challenges in the field of dementia, and musculoskeletal health. Often with multimorbidity comes polypharmacy and its consequences. Once an older person gets unwell, they need to get back to their premorbid heath with individualized care and rehabilitation.

We hope that this series on geriatrics will serve as a valuable resource for healthcare professionals, researchers, and students around the world, and that it will contribute to the ongoing effort to improve the health and well-being of older adults everywhere.

I am pleased to introduce this volume and the subsequent volumes as the Editor-in-Chief. I thank the individual volume editors and the staff of Springer Nature for their support.

Balakrishnan R. Nair

Contents

Healthy Ageing and Healthy Life Expectancy

1

Julie Byles

1.1 What Matters for Healthy Ageing?

In considering "What matters for healthy ageing?" we must ask "what matters to whom?" The answers may be very different considering older people themselves, health care providers, industry, governments, or scientists.

In this set of volumes, we have considered:

1. **Mind**—maintaining mental activity, mental state (including cognitive decline, dementia, and delirium), and mental health
2. **Mobility**—the ability to get around
3. **Multimorbidity**—the multiple pathologies that might affect people as they age
4. **Medications**—which might help or hinder older people's wellbeing
5. and what "**Matters Most**"

All of these aspects are important for improving older people's quality of life.

Intriguingly, what matters most to older people themselves has not always been the main focus of ageing programmes or research, with discourse, policy and practice often premised upon structural ageing of the population, burden of disease, dependency ratios, care requirements, and other, often negative, constructs of ageing and their effects on society.

J. Byles (✉)
School of Medicine and Public Health, The University of Newcastle,
Newcastle, NSW, Australia
e-mail: julie.byles@newcastle.edu.au

J. Byles (ed.), *What Matters for Healthy Ageing*, Topics in Geriatric Care,
https://doi.org/10.1007/978-981-96-0462-3_1

1.2 Structural Ageing

Population ageing is of course one of the most predictable and consequential global changes, not to be overtaken by other urgent concerns such as climate change, pandemics, and political disruption. Rather, ageing and older people must be part of the consideration of these issues, impacts, and solutions. Moreover, population ageing is not just a matter of people living longer, and therefore getting older. Indeed, structural ageing is largely driven by lower fertility rates, better infant and child survival, and better survival into and through adult life. You don't live up to 90 if you don't survive childhood.

Figure 1.1 shows the changes in the world population structure from 1950 to 2019 to 2050. Globally, the number of people aged 65 years and older increased from 327.6 million in 1990 to 673.7 million in 2017 [1]. In the future, the number of people aged 65 years and older is expected to rise from 0.7 billion (9%) worldwide in 2019 to 1.5 billion (16%) in 2050 [2].

1.3 Life Expectancy

Over recent decades, many countries and populations have seen an increase in life expectancy at older ages. However, the global trend towards increasing life expectancy is not inevitable or irreversible. Over the last decade, 20 out of 23 Organisation for Economic Co-operation and Development (OECD) countries have seen a reduction in the rate of increase in life expectancy. Moreover, a reduction in life expectancy has occurred in Iceland and the USA [3].

Why would this decrease in life expectancy occur in our modern developed world? The reasons are manifold including some specific causes such as maternal mortality and drug deaths (e.g. in the USA) [4]. More generally, some of the successes in mortality delay such as prevention of cardiovascular deaths have spent their main gains, and further gains in life expectancy are not forthcoming [5]. Basically, we gained a spurt in longevity through major medical breakthroughs in prevention and management of cardiovascular disease, widespread use of preventive medicines (e.g. antihypertensives and cholesterol lowering drugs, and drugs for diabetes control), and massive reductions in smoking. Against these gains, we have now added to mortality risk through increasing rates of obesity and sedentary behaviour [6].

On top of these longer term trends, COVID-19 will likely result in measurable declines in life expectancy for current cohorts now due to deaths, and in the future due to the longer term effects of the infection. In one study, life expectancy at birth declined from 2019 to 2020 in 27 out of 29 countries. The largest losses were observed for males in the USA and Lithuania (2.2 and 1.7 years, respectively). However, reductions of more than 1 year were documented in 11 countries for males and 8 countries for females. Losses were mostly due to increased mortality among

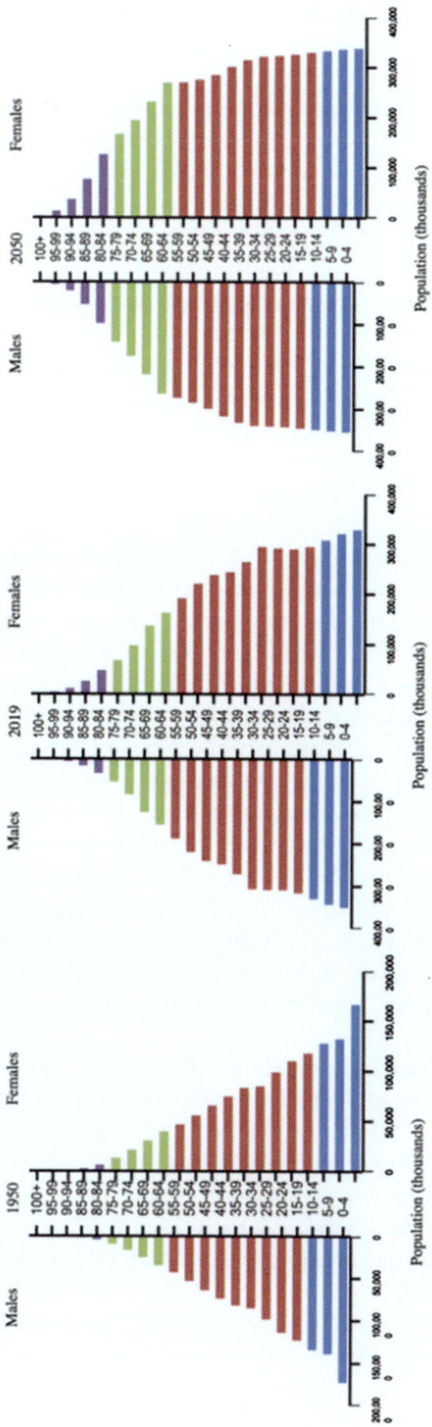

Fig. 1.1 World population structure by age and sex 1950, 2019, 2050. (Source: https://population.un.org/ProfilesOfAgeing2019/index.html)

people 60 years or over and attributed to official COVID-19 deaths [7]. These COVID-19 related losses will be even greater as the full effects of the pandemic unfold [8].

Gains in life expectancy are not uniform across all segments of the population. The differences are observed across countries, between regions within countries, and even from one end of a city to another. The differences occur by gender, ethnic and cultural group, and by social background. Low socio-economic status, adversity in childhood and adulthood, adverse health behaviours and poor mental health contribute to reduced life expectancy. Across European Union countries, the difference in life expectancy for 30-year-old men with less than higher secondary education and those with a tertiary education (a university degree or the equivalent) is around 8 years. For women the difference between higher and lower education is about 4 years [9].

1.4 Healthy Life Expectancy

While some people may be living longer, not all these years may be in good health. Health expectancies provide population health indicators combining information on health and mortality, represented as the number of years expected to be lived in good health at a particular age. Commonly these expectancies might be based on measures of self-rated health (healthy life expectancy) or the absence of disability (disability-free life expectancy). Promisingly, health expectancies have been increasing alongside increases in life expectancies, and sometimes with a relative increase in healthy years representing compression of morbidity. However, inequalities in healthy life expectancy are common and sometimes increasing, as some segments of the population gain health assets, and others lose them or fall behind.

In the United Kingdom, over the 20-year period between 1991 and 2011, healthy life expectancy at age 65 increased by 3.8 years for men and by 3.1 years for women [10], compared to increases in life expectancy of 4.5 years for men and 3.6 years for women. Since life expectancy increased proportionally more than healthy life expectancy, there was a net increase in years spent in poor health (expansion of morbidity).

Another study using data from multiple older cohorts in Australia compared the impacts of two main risk factors for poor health, obesity and smoking, on disability-free life expectancy. The study found that people in the obese BMI range were living as long as healthy weight counterparts but with more years with disability. Reducing obesity would lead to an absolute reduction of disability, especially in women. High educated obese non-smoking women living 1.3 years less than non-smoking, not obese women, but with 5.1 years fewer free of mobility disability and an extra 3.5 years with mobility disability at age 65. Men and women who smoked but were not obese lived around 2.5 years less and 2 years fewer free of disability, compared to non-smokers [11].

Another study, using data from the Australian Longitudinal Study on Women's Health, following women from age 70 to their mid 90 s. From age 70–75, the predicted length of life without disease and disability was 7·68 (CI: 7·52–7·80) years. Life with chronic disease but no disability was 4·39 (CI = 4·23–4·49) years, and life with disability was 3.76 (CI = 3·66–3·92) years. Difficulties managing on available income (HR = 1·18, 95%CI = 1·02–1·38), did not completed secondary school (HR = 1·19, 95%CI = 1·03–1·37), and overweight/obese (HR = 1·36, 95%CI = 1·20–1·55) were associated with an increased risk of disability [12].

These studies show that increases in healthy life expectancy are possible but are highly dependent on social circumstances and risk factors throughout life.

1.5 Multimorbidity and Disease Burden

Ageing is commonly associated with increased risk of disease. Population ageing is concomitantly associated with increased disease burden, expressed as Disability Adjusted Life Years (a metric that combines years of life lost to death and years of life lost to disability). Using data from the Global Burden of Disease (GBD) study, 92 GBD causes have been associated with ageing including ischaemic heart disease, intracerebral haemorrhage, other cardiovascular diseases, neoplasms, sense organ disorders, and chronic obstructive pulmonary disease. Combining data for these age-related conditions to create a metric of age-related disease burden for different countries, allows for countries to be benchmarked against the global average burden for people aged 65 years. Stacking countries up against this standard, the oldest equivalent age country was Japan, where people aged 76 years had the same disease burden as the global average 65 year old. In comparison, an average 45 year old in Papua New Guinea would have the same age-related disease burden as the global average 65 year old [13]. This fascinating study shows the wide disparity in the experience of ageing across the globe, expressed as burden of disease. It also shows that chronological age is not a constant in terms of biological age or disease burden.

Ageing is universal, but it is not uniform (Fig. 1.2).

1.6 Successful Ageing

Disease and age-associated pathological processes are a major threat to people's intrinsic capacity. In 1984, Rowe and Kahn described a state of "successful ageing", being the maintenance of physical and cognitive wellbeing in later life, with no disease or disability and high levels of engagement in life including productive activities and interpersonal relations. This premium state was in contrast with "usual ageing" where people had higher risk and disability, and "pathological ageing" where people were affected by major diseases. This construct of successful ageing has been applied in numerous research studies to identify preventive approaches to age-associated disease and disability [14, 15].

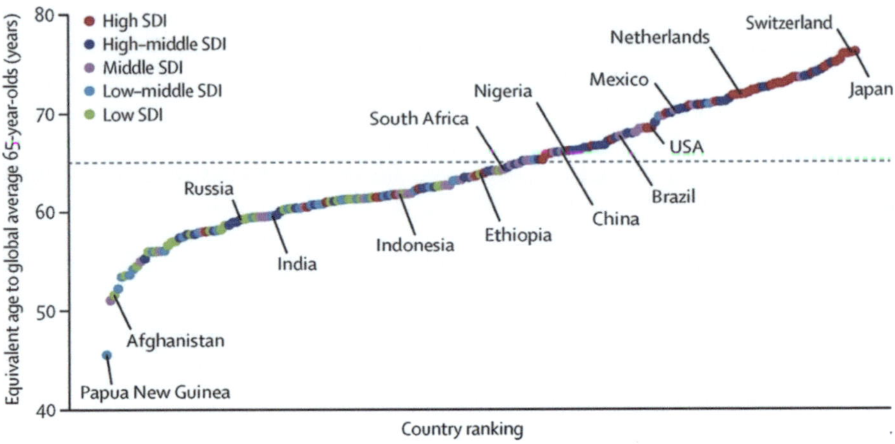

Fig. 1.2 Comparing the equivalent ages to global average 65-year-olds across countries in 2017. (Source: The Lancet Public Health, Volume 4, Issue 3, 2019)

However, what is apparent from these studies is that most people will not meet the criteria for "successful ageing". Depending on the population, the prevalence of successful ageing among people aged 65 years and over is generally estimated at less than 20%. Based on these low prevalence's, researchers consider the strict definition of successful ageing to be too narrow and to set unrealistic and unachievable expectations of older populations. A further limitation of the successful ageing definition is the inherent irony that successful ageing is less likely to apply to the very old, who may be considered the most successful given mortality selection and extended longevity.

While the concept of successful ageing presents an optimistic approach to ageing, and something to strive for, it has also attracted a wide range of criticism. Against the idea of successful ageing, many have argued that the concept is too restrictive, and that people can have enjoyment of life in older age even with some level of disease and disability. Moreover, it is argued that many older people themselves would consider themselves to have aged successfully even if they did not meet the more stringent definition of being disease and disability-free [16].

The discrepancy between the objective operationalization of successful ageing and the subjective perspective of successful ageing as expressed by older people is known as the ageing paradox. In older people's terms, success may also be defined as adapting to loss and adversity, rather than avoiding it, with the emphasis here being on the process of adaptation and coping with age-associated changes. In contrast, the objective concept of successful ageing was seen as focusing more on the outcome, rather than the process of ageing well. An alternative paradigm to successful ageing, selective optimization and compensation (SOC) [17] describes a process by which individuals compensate for losses and limitations by focusing on a small number of goals and concentrating their energy and strength in those domains. Unlike the Rowe and Kahn definition, SOC does not identify strict criteria for ageing well but emphasizes adaptive capacity with many different trajectories being identified as successful depending on the individuals' circumstances.

Other arguments against successful ageing as a construct, concern the focus on the individual and their intrinsic capacities, rather than considering the individual within the context of their environment. A neoliberal interpretation of the dominant successful ageing paradigm would see the moral responsibility for successful ageing resting with the individual relieving the state of responsibility to provide supports for older people with chronic conditions and/or disability, marginalizing older people and diminishing access to effective care, aids and other supports [18]. The concept of successful ageing could be used to drive a narrative whereby older people are expected to take personal and active control of their ageing, remain fit and youthful, contribute to the economy, and minimize demands on health and welfare [19].

The emphasis on successful ageing as a premium outcome was also criticized for not taking account of social inequalities and structural issues which increase the risks of age-related disease and disability. Many factors associated with successful ageing are beyond the control of the individual including socio-economic disadvantage, ethnicity, class, and gender. The categorical notion of "successful" and "usual" ageing also ignores the heterogeneity across the older population as well as the needs of specific sub-groups. Rowe and Khan themselves implored researchers to investigate the heterogeneity between older people, and gerontologists widely advocate for greater research on the intersection between individual and social factors that affect how people age, with "new paradigms … that more fully reflect the lived experiences of older adults" that are informed by the integration of empirical and qualitative evidence that accounts for older peoples' views [16]. This recognition of the importance of older peoples' own experiences harks back to Havighurst's original concept of successful ageing which accounted for older peoples' opinions as to what aspects of their lives were important, their own ratings of "success" as a value judgement, and highlighting the importance of adaptive processes [20].

1.7 Healthy Ageing

As we have seen in the previous sections, the later period of life is often measured in terms of increasing burden of disease and disability. However, over recent decades, there has also been an emphasis on compression of morbidity towards the end of life, and the potential for people to age "successfully" without major disease or disability and "productively" maintaining their contributions to society.

Taking these ideas a step further, the WHO 2015 World Report on Ageing and Health framed a public health goal of "healthy ageing" as a "process of developing and maintaining the functional ability that enables well-being in older age" [21].

This process of healthy ageing extends beyond notions of successful ageing which have focused on an individual remaining disease free and maintaining high levels of function and is instead centred on achieving overall wellbeing. This process of healthy ageing includes limiting the impact of disease, protecting against loss of intrinsic capacity, as well as recognizing, adapting to and supporting these needs when they arise. As such, healthy ageing represents a dynamic interaction between a person's intrinsic capacity (a person's internal strengths) and the support provided by their extrinsic social and physical environment. The balance between these factors will change over time and with age, with different trajectories of physical capacity arising depending on the balance between adversity, resistance, reserves, and other resources. The overall goal of healthy ageing is to maximize and maintain the person's functional capacity to do what they choose to do and have reason to value.

This concept of healthy ageing draws on ideas proposed by Baltes and Baltes (1990) [22] which acknowledged the balance of age-related losses and actualization of an individual's remaining strengths across the later life course through "selection, optimization and compensation". The concept of healthy ageing also changes late life goals from ageing without disease or disability, to an emphasis on overall wellbeing considering not only the person's health state, but also their capacity for community participation and social interaction, and enjoyment. Healthy ageing is inclusive of people with different levels of need, allowing for management of chronic illness, and access to care in later life (see Fig. 1.3).

WHO identified five components of functional ability to be considered in later life: the abilities to move around, meet basic needs, learn grow and make decisions, build and maintain relationships and to contribute. By enabling these abilities healthy ageing is a "freedom" that enables older people to be productive and valuable members of their communities, and not simply a burden. However, the WHO model emphasizes that the role a person may choose in later life should be decided by them and not the state or other actor, and so draws on capabilities theory [23] to frame healthy ageing around the functional ability to be and to do the things people have reason to value. The ultimate goal of healthy ageing is wellbeing and this encompasses role and identity, relationships, enjoyment, autonomy, security, and potential for personal growth.

Given that the process of ageing starts in utero and continues throughout life, healthy ageing will be affected by genetic factors, childhood conditions, health behaviours and risks in adult life, as well as the management of disease, and support for disability in later years. People will enter old age already on different paths with different levels of capacity, different threats to their health, and different levels of intrinsic reserve. Social position and personal resources will also affect how people are able to adapt to change and be supported in their older age. The concept of resilience in older age, that people can experience adversity and bounce back, is an important dynamic of healthy ageing and is against more simplistic notions of continual loss and decline. For instance, large cohort studies have shown that decline in physical capacity can reverse as well as progress [24]. Moreover, intrinsic capacity

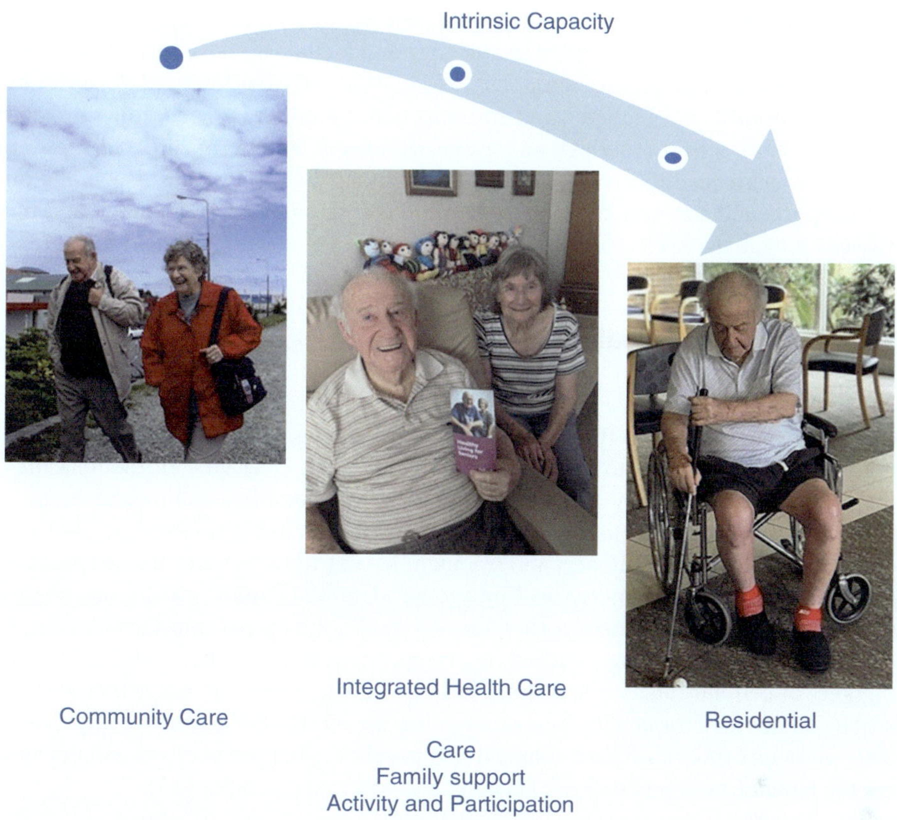

Fig. 1.3 Balancing care against declines in intrinsic capacity. (Source: Byles, J)

is moderated by multiple extrinsic environmental factors which can exacerbate limitations (if bad) or compensate for existing losses and protect against future losses (if supportive). For example, physical environments can either protect or expose people to injury throughout the life course and can encourage or hinder mobility and physical activity. Social environments can encourage and enable engagement and participation, promote emotional wellbeing, and have an impact on health behaviours. Economic and political environments govern access to resources, health care, and other supports in older age.

In a holistic life course approach to healthy ageing, frailty and need for care are not the antithesis of wellbeing, but represent separate states of risk and need. Frailty is a state of risk defined by accumulated deficits, with two widely accepted alternative definitions operationalized as a physical phenotype [25] or the accumulation of deficits in multiple domains [26, 27]. Both definitions give rise to vulnerability, and the natural history and associated outcomes of frailty are important for individual and global health [28].

Need for care includes the reliance on others for activities of daily living. Lower levels of dependency are common in older age and include need for help with higher order tasks such as transport, shopping, and cooking. Higher levels of dependency are less common and include need for help with mobility, hygiene, toileting, and transfers. Even a frail older person, or one who needs long-term care and support, can still experience more or less positive healthy ageing trajectories depending on the supports and services available to them, the environments they inhabit and the choices they make [21].

1.8 Assessing Healthy Ageing

Factors strongly predictive of healthy ageing are listed in Table 1.1. A recent systematic review identified 105 studies of healthy ageing, with most studies using a common set of domains to assess healthy ageing [29]. Over 90% of the measures included physical capacity and functioning, half included participation and engagement, half included measures of wellbeing, a quarter included personal psychological resources such as resilience, and 6% included extrinsic factors such as finances. Another review of markers for healthy ageing identified chronic conditions, cognitive decline, obesity, sarcopenia (low muscle mass), dynapenia (muscle weakness), pain, diet and nutrition, physical activity, sleep, environmental stress, and biological markers of cellular function and stress [30]. A global consortium has achieved consensus on markers for healthy ageing, creating the ATHLOS Healthy Ageing Scale. This scale incorporates both biological and psychological perspectives and considers the balance between intrinsic capacity and external resources [31].

1.9 Predicting Healthy Ageing

Longitudinal studies have shown that it is possible to assess individuals and predict their probable future trajectories of *Healthy Ageing* [30]. Analyses of data from the *Australian Longitudinal Study on Women's Health* [31], identified five distinct health-related quality of life trajectories as women age from their 70s through to

Table 1.1 Factors associated with optimal trajectories of healthy ageing across different studies

Personal Factors	Intrinsic capacity	Conditions	Functional abilities	Lifestyle	Environment
Education	Grip strength Walk speed Chair stands	Multimorbidity score BMI Muscle mass Blood pressure Biological markers	ADL IADL Cognition Mental Health	Diet Physical Activity Smoking Alcohol Social interaction	Disease management Medications Aids Social support Care

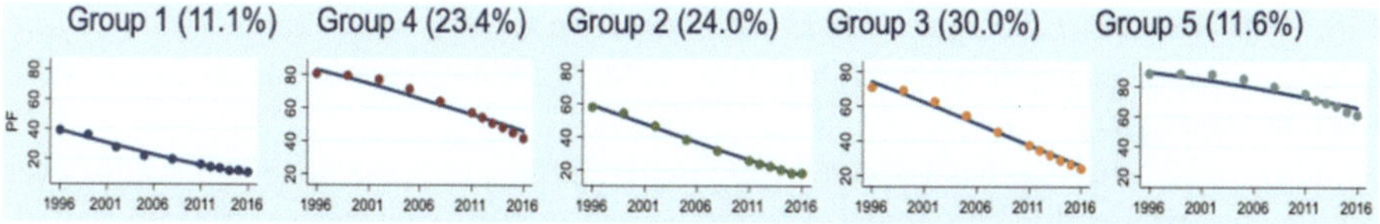

Fig. 1.4 Physical functioning trajectories (from joint trajectory models of healthy ageing). (Source: Rahman et al. Australian Longitudinal Study on Women's Health)

their 90s. These trajectories are based on the various changes in physical functioning (shown in Fig. 1.4), social functioning, mental health, bodily pain, general health, and vitality. Over this 20-year period of their lives, 12% of the women had consistently high health on all these indicators until age 90–95, with a moderate decline in physical functioning in their later years (Group 5). However, 11% of women had poor and declining health in terms of physical functioning, general health, bodily pain, and vitality from age 70–75, while still maintaining a moderate but declining social functioning and mental health until age 82–87 (Group 1). Groups 2–4 had moderate or good health at the start of observation, but then various rates of decline as they aged.

Similarly, an analysis of 16 years of data from the Melbourne Longitudinal Studies in Healthy Ageing identified three trajectories of ageing well: "stable and ageing well" (30.2% women, 28% of men); "initially ageing well then deteriorating" (50.5% of women and 47.6% of men); and "stable and ageing poorly" (19.3% women and 24.4% men). Factors associated with poorer trajectories included personal characteristics such as level of education and socio-economic status, health behaviours such as smoking and physical activity, body mass index (underweight or overweight/obese), good nutrition, chronic conditions, restful sleep, decreased strain, and social support [32].

Many other longitudinal studies have established risk profiles for people at risk of functional decline, finding a similar range of personal and lifestyle predictors. In these studies, education, income and other sociodemographic factors are often a critical element in determining how well people will age [33–40]. These factors are in turn related to both health risk behaviours and access to quality health care, and many factors may be modifiable in later life [37]. These lifestyle factors which include nutrition, physical activity, alcohol, and smoking have been found to be strongly associated with later life outcomes such as successful ageing [41–44], functional decline [36, 45], wellbeing [35, 46], healthy ageing [47, 48], disability-free life expectancy, and healthy life expectancy [11, 49, 50]. There is also some evidence that social factors such as social engagement and support may play a role [37]. For example, in a recent analysis of data from over 11,000 men and women from six countries in Europe, healthy lifestyle and psychosocial indicators were strongly associated with measures of healthy ageing. For men aged 60–67, the odds of healthy ageing increased by 32.5% with each point increase in the lifestyle index

(18.7% for women). Similar odds ratios were seen for ages 68–79, and effects were stronger for those aged 80 years or over. Effects for the psychosocial index were even stronger [37].

These and other studies form a strong evidence-base for the development of predictive algorithms that characterize probable and possible pathways for ageing well, depending on an individual's risk profile.

1.10 Mortality Rates and Survivor Effects

The health of a cohort of people will change with mortality rates, and as people with higher rates of disease and disability die and leave the cohort. This effect, known as mortality selection, can result in a relatively healthy and robust cohort of people at older ages [51]. However, at extreme old ages there is a deceleration in mortality, regardless of the level of frailty, and the dynamic effects of mortality selection on the cohort may not be as apparent. Moreover, selection effects do not occur equally or contemporaneously across all social groups, with the effect on the total cohort depending on effects within sub-groups defined by socio-economic status, disease, or other factors that can have an impact on both disability and rate of death.

1.11 Healthy Ageing and Longevity—Approaching 100

Centenarians are often considered to be a "model of ageing well" as people who have lived long and avoided or delayed the onset of disease and disability until much later in life [52]. Around the world, there has been increasing recognition of the importance of characterizing the phenotype and genotype of people who live beyond 95 years with potential to become centenarians or even super centenarians [53]. Studies of centenarians as successful agers have classified people as "escapers" who have no chronic age-associated diseases, "delayers" who developed disease after age 80, and "survivors" who have lived to very old age despite earlier disease onset. For example, the Georgia Ageing Study, classified 32% of their centenarians as escapers, 36% as delayers, and 43% as survivors. There were two main clusters of conditions affecting these older people: one involving cancer (major onset in 60s), CVD (major onset in 70s), anaemia, and osteoporosis and another associated with dementia (major onset in 80s) [54].

1.12 What Matters Most to Older People

Older age is a challenging time for many people, they face increasing complexities of disease, they may have declining cognitive and physical capacity, and their social and physical environments may not be optimal to support their needs. How do older people weigh up this balance between increasing needs and diminishing resources, to find joy and satisfaction in their later lives? In these volumes, we have followed the rule of the "5Ms". In considering what matters most we have applied the healthy ageing frame, where the goal is to maintain people's abilities to be and do what they choose to do and have reason to value. These activities might include functioning, enjoying life, connecting, and managing health [55]. In one study of 105 older people attending outpatient clinics at Veterans Affairs' Medical Center in Boston, Massachusetts were interviewed to identify their values in relation to health care decisions. Their priority values included taking care of themselves, thinking about things clearly, mobility and living at home. They wanted to enjoy hobbies and relationships with family and friends, without being a burden to others. In terms of health, they wanted to avoid pain and discomfort, with quality of life having priority over length of life [56].

Another window into what matters to older people may be provided by interviews with women from the Australian Longitudinal Study on Women's Health who had survived to their mid to late 90s. Most women recognized the effects of ageing on their body and their intrinsic capacity, and that they were "slowing down a bit". However, there was a sense of acceptance that physical limitations and health problems were a part of life, and normal for their age, and so they just got on with things. There was also a strong theme of resilience and resourcefulness in the women's abilities to adapt and to use support systems to continue to live a fulfilled life. The activities women engaged in ranged from relatively passive individual pursuits such as reading or sewing, to social activities such as cards, to strong engagement and purpose in family and communities. Puzzles such as sudoku and crosswords were also activities that women enjoyed on their own within their own homes. Many women engaged in these mental activities for amusement and enjoyment, but others saw them as a way of retaining their mental capacities. Knitting, sewing, and craft were also popular activities, some women crocheting for charities or the homeless. For many women, continuing to be productive, cooking, keeping busy and engaged in life were paramount to feeling connected and useful, and gave life meaning. They found satisfaction in completing housework or other activities of daily living. The majority of women had a high priority for social activities, including outings with friends. Many of the women continued to drive themselves. For these women, driving was important not only for transport, but also for autonomy and identity. Family was a strong theme throughout the interviews, which brought much happiness, and ongoing community participation was also important. Many took joy in remembering, and in "just being" [57].

1.13 Conclusion

Ageing is a pervasive construct with multiple perspectives. At a basic level ageing is the ticking of the clock, adding to life's timeline from birth to death. But chronological age is far from the most important matter, with factors such as intrinsic capacity, identity, activity, and support mattering far more. The ancient Greeks had two words for time, *Chronos*—a quantitative measure, the ticking of the clock; and *Kairos*—a qualitative measure of the moments [58]. For older people, moments may be more important than minutes (Box 1.1).

Box 1.1 A Conceptualization of Healthy Ageing for Women in Their 90s

Wellbeing	
Identity To be what you value	
Activities + Participation To do what you value	
Intrinsic Capacity	**Supportive Environments**
Body systems and function	Social connection
Health conditions	Social support
Instrumental/Activities of Daily. Living (IADL/ADL)	Informal instrumental support
Cognition	Formal services
Mental Health	Housing and Built environments
Internal resources	Aids and devices
Personal factors	Finance

Source: Byles et al. Australian Longitudinal Study on Women's Health [57]

References

1. Cheng X, Yang Y, Schwebel DC, Liu Z, Li L, Cheng P, Ning P, Hu G. Population ageing and mortality during 1990–2017: a global decomposition analysis. PLoS Med. 2020;17(6):e1003138.
2. Population Division. World Population Prospects 2019. Geneva: United Nations, Department of Social and Economic Affairs; 2019. https://population.un.org/wpp/Publications/Files/wpp2019_10KeyFindings.pdf. Accessed 27 Jan 2022.
3. Ho JY, Hendi AS. Recent trends in life expectancy across high income countries: retrospective observational study. BMJ. 2018;362:k2562. https://doi.org/10.1136/bmj.k2562.
4. Harper S, Riddell CA, King NB. Declining life expectancy in the United States: missing the trees for the forest. Annu Rev Public Health. 2021;42:381–403. https://doi.org/10.1146/annurev-publhealth-082619-104231. Epub 2021 Dec 16.
5. Mehta NK, Abrams LR, Myrskylä M. US life expectancy stalls due to cardiovascular disease, not drug deaths. Proc Natl Acad Sci U S A. 2020;117(13):6998–7000.
6. Crimmins EM. Recent trends and increasing differences in life expectancy present opportunities for multidisciplinary research on aging. Nat Aging. 2021;1:12–3.
7. Aburto JM, Schöley J, Kashnitsky I, Zhang L, Rahal C, Missov TI, Mills MC, Dowd JB, Kashyap R. Quantifying impacts of the COVID-19 pandemic through life-expectancy losses: a population-level study of 29 countries. Int J Epidemiol. 2022;51(1):63–74.
8. Schöley J, Aburto JM, Kashnitsky I, Kniffka MS, Zhang L, Jaadla H, Dowd JB, Kashyap R. Life expectancy changes since COVID-19. Nat Hum Behav. 2022 Dec;6(12):1649–59.
9. OECD. Inequalities in life expectancy. Health at a Glance: Europe 2018: State of Health in the EU Cycle. Paris: OECD Publishing; 2018.

10. Jagger C, Matthews FE, Wohland P, Fouweather T, Stephan BC, Robinson L, Arthur A, Brayne C. A comparison of health expectancies over two decades in England: results of the Cognitive Function and Ageing Study I and II. Lancet. 2016;387(10020):779–86.
11. Kingston A, Byles J, Kiely K, Anstey KJ, Jagger C. The impact of smoking and obesity on disability-free life expectancy in older Australians. J Gerontol A Biol Sci Med Sci. 2021;76(7):1265–72. https://doi.org/10.1093/gerona/glaa290.
12. Md Rahman M, Jagger C; Princehorn EM, Holliday EG, Leigh L, Loxton D, Beard J, Byles JE, Kowal P. Predicting chronic disease, disability and mortality in a large cohort of older australian women: A markov multi-state modelling approach. Available at SSRN: https://ssrn.com/abstract=3821481 or https://doi.org/10.2139/ssrn.3821481.
13. Chang AY, Skirbekk VF, Tyrovolas S, Kassebaum NJ, Dieleman JL. Measuring population ageing: an analysis of the Global Burden of Disease Study 2017. Lancet Pub Health. 2019;4(3):e159–67.
14. Urtamo A, Jyväkorpi SK, Strandberg TE. Definitions of successful ageing: a brief review of a multidimensional concept. Acta Biomed. 2019;90(2):359–63.
15. Lafortune L, Martin S, Kelly S, Kuhn I, Remes O, Cowan A, Brayne C. Behavioural risk factors in mid-life associated with successful ageing, disability, dementia and frailty in later life: a rapid systematic review. PLoS One. 2016;11(2):e0144405.
16. Martinson M, Berridge C. Successful aging and its discontents: a systematic review of the social gerontology literature. Gerontologist. 2015;55(1):58–69. https://doi.org/10.1093/geront/gnu037.
17. Baltes B, Dickson MW. Using life-span models in industrial-organizational psychology: The theory of selective optimization with compensation. Appl Dev Sci. 2001;5(1):51–62.
18. Rubinstein RL, de Medeiros K. "Successful aging," gerontological theory and neoliberalism: a qualitative critique. Gerontologist. 2015;55(1):34–42.
19. Katz S, Calasanti T. Critical perspectives on successful aging: does it "appeal more than it illuminates"? Gerontologist. 2015;55(1):26–33.
20. Havighurst RJ. Successful aging. Gerontologist. 1961;1(1):8–13.
21. World Health Organization. World report on ageing and health. Geneva: World Health Organization; 2015.
22. Baltes PB, Baltes MM. Psychological perspectives on successful aging: the model of selective optimization with compensation. In: Baltes PB, Baltes MM, editors. Successful aging: perspectives from the behavioral sciences. Cambridge: Cambridge University Press; 1990. p. 1–34.
23. Sen A. Human rights and capabilities. Hum Dev. 2006;6(2):151–66.
24. Qualls C, Waters DL, Vellas B, Villareal DT, Garry PJ, Gallini A, Andrieu S. Reversible states of physical and/or cognitive dysfunction: a 9-Year longitudinal study. J Nutr Health Aging. 2017;21(3):271–5.
25. Fried LP, Ferrucci L, Darer J, Williamson JD, Anderson G. Untangling the concepts of disability, frailty and comorbidity: implications for improved targeting and care. J Gerontol A Biol Sci Med Sci. 2004;59(3):255–63.
26. Mitnitski A, Mogilner A, Rockwood K. Accumulation of deficits as a proxy measure of aging. Sci World J. 2001;1:323–36.
27. Rockwood K, Mitnitski A. Frailty defined by deficit accumulation and geriatric medicine defined by frailty. Clin Geriatr Med. 2011;27(1):17–26.
28. Rodriguez-Artalejo F, Rodriguez-Manas L. The frailty syndrome in the public health agenda. J Epidemiol Community Health. 2014;0:1–2.
29. Cosco TD, Prina AM, Perales J, Stephan BC, Brayne C. Operational definitions of successful aging: a systematic review. Int Psychogeriatr. 2014;26(3):373–81.
30. Anton SD, Woods AJ, Ashizawa T, Barb D, Buford TW, Carter CS, et al. Successful aging: advancing the science of physical independence in older adults. Ageing Res Rev. 2015;24:304–27.
31. Sanchez-Niubo A, et al. Development of a common scale for measuring healthy ageing across the world: results from the ATHLOS consortium. Int J Epidemiol. 2021;50(3):880–92.

32. Browning CJ, Enticott JC, Thomas SA, Kendig H. Trajectories of ageing well among older Australians: a 16-year longitudinal study. Ageing Soc. 2018;38(8):1581–602.
33. Leigh L, Byles JE, Mishra GD. Change in physical function among women as they age: findings from the Australian Longitudinal Study on Women's Health. Qual Life Res. 2017;26(4):981–91.
34. Rahman MM, Byles JE, et al. Healthy Ageing Trajectories from the Australian Longitudinal Study on Women's Health [Unpublished], 2022.
35. Kendig H, Loh V, O'Loughlin K, Byles J, Nazroo JY. Pathways to well-being in later life: socioeconomic and health determinants across the life course of Australian Baby Boomers. J Popul Ageing. 2016;9:49–67.
36. Chatterji S, Byles J, Cutler D, Seeman T, Verdes E. Health, functioning, and disability in older adults—present status and future implications. Lancet. 2015;385(9967):563–75.
37. Sowa A, Tobiasz-Adamczyk B, Topór-Mądry R, Poscia A, la Milia DI. Predictors of healthy ageing: public health policy targets. BMC Health Serv Res. 2016;16 Suppl 5(Suppl 5):289.
38. Etman A, Burdorf A, Van der Cammen TJ, Mackenbach JP, Van Lenthe FJ. Socio-demographic determinants of worsening in frailty among community-dwelling older people in 11 European countries. J Epidemiol Community Health. 2012;66(12):1116–21.
39. Ovrum A, Gustavsen GW, Rickertsen K. Age and socioeconomic inequalities in health: examining the role of lifestyle choices. Adv Life Course Res. 2014;19:1–13.
40. Sanchez-Niubo A, Egea-Cortés L, Olaya B, Caballero FF, Ayuso-Mateos JL, Prina M, Bobak M, Arndt H, Tobiasz-Adamczyk B, Pająk A, Leonardi M, Koupil I, Panagiotakos D, Tamosiunas A, Scherbov S, Sanderson W, Koskinen S, Chatterji S, Haro JM, ATHLOS Consortium. Cohort Profile: The Ageing Trajectories of Health—Longitudinal Opportunities and Synergies (ATHLOS) project. Int J Epidemiol. 2019;48(4):1052–1053i. https://doi.org/10.1093/ije/dyz077.
41. Ward M, McGarrigle CA, Kenny RA. More than health: quality of life trajectories among older adults—findings from The Irish Longitudinal Study of Ageing (TILDA). Qual Life Res. 2019;28:429–39. https://doi.org/10.1007/s11136-018-1997-y.
42. Anton SD, Woods AJ, Ashizawa T, Barb D, Buford TW, Carter CS, Clark DJ, Cohen RA, Corbett DB, Cruz-Almeida Y, Dotson V, Ebner N, Efron PA, Fillingim RB, Foster TC, Gundermann DM, Joseph AM, Karabetian C, Leeuwenburgh C, Manini TM, Marsiske M, Mankowski RT, Mutchie HL, Perri MG, Ranka S, Rashidi P, Sandesara B, Scarpace PJ, Sibille KT, Solberg LM, Someya S, Uphold C, Wohlgemuth S, Wu SS, Pahor M. Successful aging: Advancing the science of physical independence in older adults. Ageing Res Rev. 2015;24(Pt B):304–27.
43. Byles JE, Rahman MM, Princehorn EM, Holliday EG, Leigh L, Loxton D, Beard J, Kowal P, Jagger C. Successful ageing from old to very old: a longitudinal study of 12,432 women from Australia. Age Ageing. 2019;48(6):803–10.
44. Bosnes I, Nordahl HM, Stordal E, Bosnes O, Myklebust TÅ, Almkvist O. Lifestyle predictors of successful aging: a 20-year prospective HUNT study. PLoS One. 2019;14(7):e0219200.
45. Jonkman NH, Del Panta V, Hoekstra T, Colpo M, van Schoor NM, Bandinelli S, Cattelani L, Helbostad JL, Vereijken B, Pijnappels M, Maier AB. Predicting trajectories of functional decline in 60- to 70-year-old people. Gerontology. 2018;64(3):212–21.
46. Steptoe A, Deaton A, Stone AA. Subjective wellbeing, health, and ageing. Lancet. 2015;385(9968):640–8. https://doi.org/10.1016/S0140-6736(13)61489-0. Epub 2014 Nov 6.
47. Daskalopoulou C, Koukounari A, Wu YT, Terrera GM, Caballero FF, De La Fuente J, Tyrovolas S, Panagiotakos DB, Prince M, Prina M. Healthy ageing trajectories and lifestyle behaviour: the Mexican Health and Aging Study. Sci Rep. 2019;9(1):1–0.
48. Södergren M. Lifestyle predictors of healthy ageing in men. Maturitas. 2013;75(2):113–7.
49. Wubishet BL, Byles JE, Harris ML, Jagger C. Impact of diabetes on life and healthy life expectancy among older women. J Gerontol Ser A. 2021;76(5):914–21.
50. Rahman MM, Jagger C, Leigh L, Holliday E, Princehorn E, Loxton D, Kowal P, Beard J, Byles J. The impact of education and lifestyle factors on disability-free life expectancy from mid-life to older age: a multi-cohort study. Int J Public Health. 2022;67:1605045.

51. Zheng H. Aging in the context of cohort evolution and mortality selection. Demography. 2014;51(4):1295–317.
52. Borras C, Ingles M, Mas-Bargues C, Dromant M, Sanz-Ros J, Román-Domínguez A, Gimeno-Mallench L, Gambini J, Viña J. Centenarians: an excellent example of resilience for successful ageing. Mech Ageing Dev. 2020;186:111199.
53. Teo SP. A review of centenarian studies. Qeios. 2022; https://doi.org/10.32388/MFX83V.
54. Davey A, Elias MF, Siegler IC, Lele U, Martin P, Johnson MA, Hausman DB, Poon LW. Cognitive function, physical performance, health, and disease: norms from the Georgia centenarian study. Exp Aging Res. 2010;36(4):394–425.
55. Tinetti M, Naik A, Dindo L. Conversation guide for patients and caregivers for identifying their health priorities. USA: Patient Priorities Care; 2018. https://patientprioritiescare.org/wp-content/uploads/2018/11/Conversation-Guide-and-Manual-for-Identifying-Patients27-Health-Priorities.pdf. Accessed 22 Jan 2022.
56. Moye J, Driver JA, Montgomery MP, Owsiany T, Chen LQ, Whitley JC, Auguste EJ, Paik JM. Assessing what matters most in older adults with multicomplexity. Gerontologist. 2022;60(4):e224–34.
57. Byles J, Tavener M, Princehorn E. Healthy Ageing at very old ages—perspectives from women in the oldest cohort of the Australian Longitudinal Study on Women's Health. In 'Handbook of Contemporary Ageing Issues: Global and Country Narratives' Editor: Dr. Mala Kapur Shankardass, Ph.D Routledge (in Press—due early 2023).
58. Smith JE. Time, times, and the 'Right Time'; "Chronos" And "Kairos". Monist Philos Hist. 1969;53(1):1–13.

Social and Cultural Determinants of Ageing

2

Julie Byles, Xiaoyue Xu,
and Vasoontara Sbirakos Yiengprugsawan

2.1 Introduction

The experience of ageing is determined by so much more than chronological age. In this chapter, we will look at how social and cultural factors affect how people age. What is clear is that social determinants such as education, income, and other (good and bad) life circumstances affect how people age [1]. It is also clear that these effects commence in utero, throughout childhood and early life. These foundations set the shape of a person's health and other circumstances throughout life and as they age. While it is never too late to make positive changes throughout life, the early years will always exert some effect on our later lives.

A review of social factors associated with successful ageing has identified four social domains that can exert influence on later life: sociodemographic and socioeconomic factors (considered here); social engagement, community participation, social support, and social networks and integration (considered in future Chap. 4) [1].

2.2 Socioeconomic Circumstances

Social and economic disadvantage in childhood [2–4] and midlife [5, 6] are associated with ongoing health inequalities in later life. There is an increasing interest in understanding how these life-long socioeconomic circumstances impact on the

J. Byles (✉)
School of Medicine and Public Health, The University of Newcastle,
Newcastle, NSW, Australia
e-mail: julie.byles@newcastle.edu.au

X. Xu · V. S. Yiengprugsawan
University of New South Wales, Sydney, NSW, Australia
e-mail: luna.xu@unsw.edu.au; v.yiengpr@unsw.edu.au

J. Byles (ed.), *What Matters for Healthy Ageing*, Topics in Geriatric Care,
https://doi.org/10.1007/978-981-96-0462-3_2

intrinsic and extrinsic resources and vulnerabilities accumulated course of life, and how they affect people's well-being in later life.

In considering the impacts of social factors, three models have been postulated:

- The sensitive period model, whereby early life factors predispose to a lifetime of disadvantage and poorer outcomes.
- The accumulation of risks model, whereby negative exposures and risk factors accumulate over time.
- The pathway model, whereby childhood circumstances lead to adult events, but these causal paths may be mediated by adult circumstances [7].

These three models are not necessarily mutually incompatible. For instance, early life factors, such as maternal nutrition, may be reflected in birth weight. Birth weight, in turn, has been associated with adult disease including cardiovascular disease [8] and frailty (sensitive period) [9]. Ongoing socioeconomic disadvantage in childhood may include poor nutrition, parental discord, and lower levels of education. These would lead to lower status occupations with higher risk, and ongoing social disadvantage (pathway). Across the life course risks accumulate including periods of poor mental health, smoking, drinking, poor nutrition, obesity building to a large area under the curve in terms of risk exposure (accumulation).

A number of studies have analysed life history data to determine the evidence for these different life course effects. Data from the Survey of Health, Ageing and Retirement in Europe (SHARE) provide evidence of the effects of childhood socioeconomic status on life satisfaction and quality of life for people aged 50 years and over [10]. Another analysis of data from SHARE provides further evidence for the cumulative effects of childhood socioeconomic status, as well as the mediating role of education and welfare, on quality of life in older adults [11].

In the English Longitudinal Study of Ageing, life history data has been used to understand the causal pathways between lifetime socioeconomic status and later life outcomes such as cardiovascular disease. Socioeconomic status across the life course was a strong predictor of cardiovascular mortality. People who had low socioeconomic status across their lives experienced the greatest risk. Mostly, this socioeconomic gradient in cardiovascular mortality was explained by associated variations in behavioural, psychosocial, physiological, and inflammatory risk factors [12].

Similarly, a study conducted in Newcastle Upon-Tyne in the United Kingdom, found strong positive effects of higher occupational status in mid-life and better self-reported health, employment, and mortgage-freedom in later adulthood. Social class at birth and level of education had indirect effects of quality of life, mediated through later-life socioeconomic advantage. Similar to the Australian study, the results support a pathway model with the effects of factors in earlier life acting through later-life factors, and an accumulation model with earlier-life factors having cumulative effects on quality of life at older ages. Further, a direct effect of adverse childhood events by age five on adult quality of life suggests a sensitive period with childhood effects lasting across the lifetime [13].

Other evidence suggests that socioeconomic disadvantage is associated with biomarkers of stress and activation of physiological mechanisms for age-associated chronic diseases. Lower levels of education, income, and occupational status have been associated with higher circulating levels of acute phase proteins such as C-reactive protein (CRP) and other markers of inflammation, infection, and metabolic dysregulation [14]. These effects are both direct, suggesting the sensitive stage hypothesis, and indirect with early life circumstances setting the trajectory for socioeconomic status across the life course.

Modelling on the English Longitudinal Study on Ageing, an Australian study looked at the pathways between childhood and early adult circumstances, and well-being at age 60 years (measured as life satisfaction and quality of life). Current age showed an association with life satisfaction but not quality of life, while gender not associated with either. Being married or in a de facto relationship was positively related to both well-being measures, while only quality of life was related to being in paid work. Adult socioeconomic status and health indicators generally had larger correlations with both well-being measures than the childhood indicators. The childhood factor that had a significant direct effect was the number of books at home which correlated with higher quality of life at age 60–65 years. Importantly, the study found that adult socioeconomic status mediates the effects of childhood socioeconomic status on later well-being, and adult health mediates the effects of childhood health on well-being. Moreover, consistent with the accumulation model, the number of negative socioeconomic status and health exposures across the life course was related to poorer well-being outcomes among older adults [15].

Also in the Australian Life Histories and Health Study, perceived poor parental quality was a risk for both ever and current depression for both sexes. For men, over-protective fathers were a risk for ever and current depression, while poor parental quality was a risk for reporting treatment for depression. These relative risks for current depression and treatment attenuated after controlling for current mood, but remained a significant risk for having reported a lifetime diagnosis for depression and anxiety [16].

2.3 Cultural Influences

Different cultures will have different attitudes to ageing, and hold older people in different regard, with different expectations and status. Attitudes towards ageing may be more positive in some social contexts, with popular belief that older people in eastern societies are held in higher regard than in developed western societies. Filial piety is often cited as a pillar of the position of older people in eastern societies.

Culture may also play a role in the maintenance and size of social networks as people age. These effects may play out across different countries, religions, and ethnic groups, but also across urban and rural settings [17].

The care that older people can expect to receive will also differ across cultural settings. Western societies tend to have a greater reliance on formal care services, whereas other cultures may have a greater reliance on family care, and stronger village support networks. Multigenerational households are likely to increase intergenerational interdependence [18].

Within English-speaking countries migrant elders who do not speak English may experience ageing differently to English speakers and to their counterparts who remained in their home countries. A study of the cultural determinants of health for older adults, found that those with lower English proficiency with demonstrated adherence to cultural beliefs about health and illness, differential attitudes between traditional healing practices and western medicine, and a general distrust of western health care [19]. Also, language and cultural barriers impeded their access to western health information and resources. In another study, while families played an important role, language and cultural barriers impeded older people's access to health information and resources [20].

An overview of 11 studies of lay views of healthy ageing compared western and non-western cultural perspectives and also compared the views of academics and lay older people. In general, lay definitions included more domains and more diversity in the healthy ageing concept than academic views. Whereas academic views tend to focus more on physical and mental health and social functioning in later life, the lay views considered factors such as independence, family, adaptation, financial security, personal growth, and spirituality. Comparing people from different cultural backgrounds and country settings, mental function was less likely to be mentioned in studies from Asia than in studies from Europe and Canada. Family was more commonly mentioned in Asian studies [21].

2.4 Socioeconomic Determinants of Ageing in China, a Case Study

The ageing of populations in China is an important demographic phenomenon with significant challenges and opportunities. China is a fast transitioning and diverse society that is rapidly ageing due both to low fertility rates (accelerated by the one child policy) and improved longevity. The proportion of the population aged 60 years and over will increase from 12.4% in 2010 to 28% in 2040 [22]. Women outlive men, and populations in rural areas have proportionally more older people.

In addition to this rapid demographic transition, China is also facing a rapid epidemiological transition with increasing incidence and prevalence of non-communicable ageing. This transition is partly driven by population ageing, with older people more at risk of such conditions, but is also driven with changes in lifestyle and other health risks with age-specific increases in disease burden. More than 30% of non-communicable disease burden in China is for people 60 years and over [22].

Chinese society is also changing with increased industrialization and changes to family structures. Traditionally *filial piety* has been a defining feature of Chinese society, setting norms for parent–child relationships across the life course whereby the child supports and succeeds the parent [23]. Until recently, most older Chinese

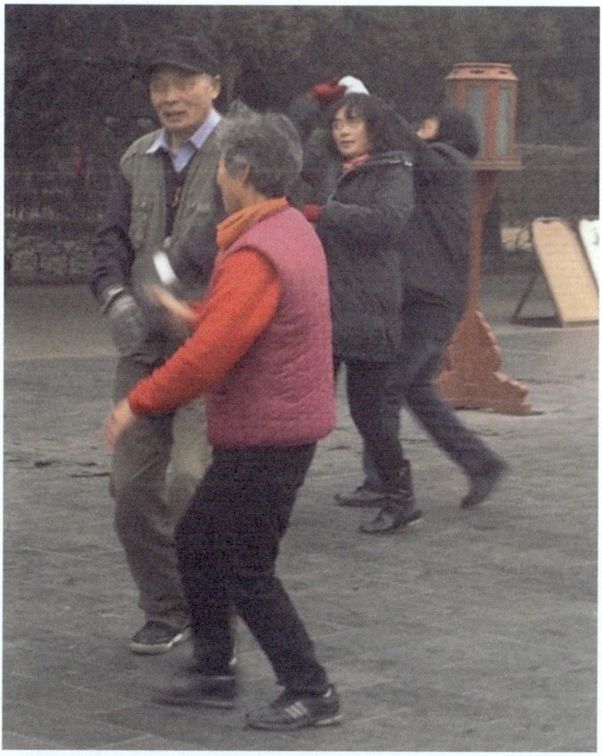

Picture 2.1 Dancing in the park. Beijing China. (Source: Byles J. Personal collection)

people lived with their son or daughter, supported by their children and grandchildren. More recently, there have been sharp declines in co-residence of older people with their families. In one study, it was estimated that 34% of people 60 years or over lived in three-generation families, 14% lived in two-generation families and the remainder did not live with their children. In this study, people with greater family care resources, more children and a living spouse, those with more economic resources, and those in urban areas, tended to prefer to not live away from their children [24] (Picture 2.1).

The current cohort of older Chinese people has lived through social change, with major economic reforms from the late 1970s and early 1980s. These changes include extensive and uneven urbanization, the one-child policy, and educational advancement. Based on data from the China Health and Retirement Longitudinal Study (CHARLS), a life course analytical study has confirmed that educational attainment, urban residence, relative living standard, and medical insurance schemes are the most important social and economic predictors of health. Notably for men, relative living standard and urban residence are the most significant while, for women, living standard and secondary schooling are the main socioeconomic determinants of health in later life [25].

2.5 Chronic Diseases Among Older People in China

China has a similar non-communicable disease profile to the rest of the world, with most deaths being attributed to stroke and ischaemic heart disease, chronic respiratory disease, diabetes, and cancers [26]. According to the Global Burden of Disease Study, between 1990 and 2017, population ageing was associated with 92.8 million disability adjusted life years (DALYs) in China. Of these, 65.8% (61.1 million) were years of life lost (YLLs). The top five causes of ageing-associated DALYs were stroke, chronic obstructive pulmonary disease, ischaemic heart disease, tracheal, bronchus, and lung cancer and liver cancer. Against this increase in DALYs, age-specific DALYs had decreased, mostly due to improvements in modifiable risk factors [27]. Between 1990 and 2017, age-specific DALY rate reductions offset DALY increases related to population ageing (−196.2 million versus +92.8 million), with 57.5% (−112.8 million) of the decrease attributed to 84 modifiable risk factors [27].

It is said that China now has the largest diabetes epidemic in the world with around 11% of the older population having diabetes in 2013 [28]. If these major diseases were eliminated, there would be significant increases in health-adjusted life expectancies [29]. While such theoretical elimination may be impossible, these diseases have common and shared behavioural risk factors which are largely modifiable through changes to lifestyle and related risk factors [30, 31].

Smoking is a major modifiable risk factor for chronic disease in China. China is the world's largest consumer of tobacco, with consequent effects on the country's chronic disease burden. An estimated 26% of Chinese adults smoke, with little reduction in overall prevalence from 2003 to 2013. For men the prevalence is 48%, compared to 4% for women [32].

2.6 Prevalence of Disability Among Older People in China

The prevalence of successful ageing is low among Chinese older people [33]. Data from the WHO Global Study of Ageing and adult health (WHO-SAGE) China were used to estimate the proportion of people aged 60 or over who were classified as having difficulty on each of eight daily living items:

- Moving around inside the house
- Walking 100 m
- Standing up from sitting down
- Getting up from lying down
- Getting to and using the toilet
- Bathing/washing whole body
- Getting dressed
- Eating

Generally, the most common difficulties were with walking 100 m (16% of people 60+), and with getting up from sitting down (17%). Getting dressed (9%) and eating (11%) were the items with the lowest prevalence of difficulty. Compared to other countries, China had the lowest prevalence of difficulty and lowest scores on disability measures [33]. It should also be considered that these difficulties do not reflect only intrinsic capacity, but may also be influenced by inadequate environmental supports or barriers. For instance, toilet facilities may vary across countries, increasing the degree of difficulty with toileting in some settings.

It is also likely that different disabilities will cluster together, with people who have difficulty on one item having difficulty on another. These disabilities will also progress along a hierarchy with higher order abilities being lost before lower order ones.

Latent Class Analysis (LCA) can be used to identify different sub-groups with similar functional difficulties (according to probabilities of class membership). Figure 2.1 shows three disability profiles for people aged 60 years or over in China, based on WHO-SAGE data. In this figure, 6% of people have difficulty on all items, 15% have difficulty on some items, and 78% had few difficulties.

For China, the class with no difficulties were the youngest, with those in the classes with few difficulties aged less than 70, and the class with difficulty on all items aged around 75. There were more women than men in the classes with disability. Most people were partnered, but those with disability were less likely to be partnered. Most had primary school education or less. Those with difficulties tended to be more in rural areas, and those with no difficulties more in urban areas (see Table 2.1).

Other analysis of data from the WHO-SAGE study for Chinese aged 50 years and older has revealed substantial geographic disparities across China in health-related outcomes and productivity, potentially reflecting structural differences in access to health care, as well as economic and cultural variation and the importance

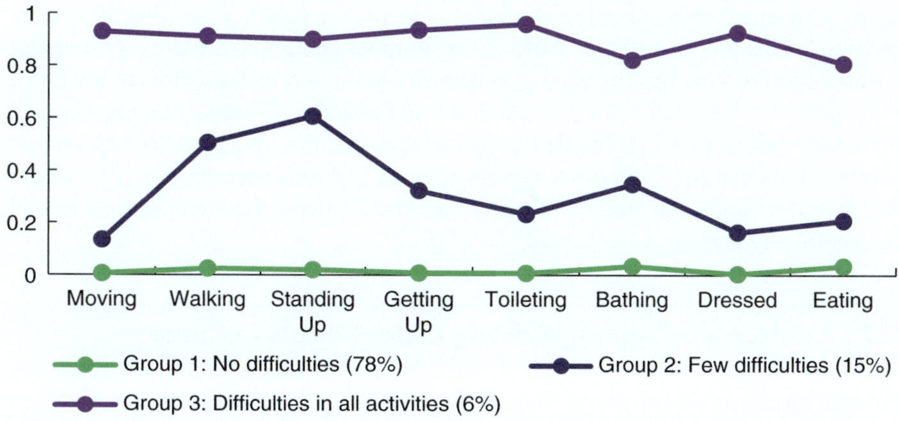

Fig. 2.1 Disability profiles for people aged 60 years or over in China. (Source: WHO-SAGE data, unpublished analyses by Byles J and Thapaliya K. 2022)

Table 2.1 Characteristics of people in each disability class

	Difficulties in all activities (6%), $N = 477$	Few difficulties (15%), $N = 918$	No difficulties (78%), $N = 5910$
Age			
Mean	74.5	72.0	68.8
Age groups	%	%	%
60–69	**29**	**38**	**58**
70–79	**43**	**45**	**35**
80 and above	**28**	**17**	**7**
Gender			
Men	**43**	**39**	**49**
Women	**57**	**61**	**51**
Marital Status			
Partnered	**68**	**69**	**78**
Non-partnered	**32**	**31**	**22**
Less than primary school	**32**	**35**	**25**
Primary school	**33**	**34**	**28**
Secondary school	**22**	**16**	**22**
High school	**9**	**11**	**16**
College and above	**4**	**4**	**9**
Area			
Urban	**40**	**43**	**55**
Rural	**60**	**57**	**45**

Source: WHO-SAGE data, unpublished analyses by Byles J and Thapaliya K. 2022

of local cultural context in informing policy and practice [30]. There were large differences between urban and rural areas observed in both the well-developed areas (e.g. Shandong) and also the lower end of the economic spectrum (e.g. Hubei and Jilin). Covariates significantly associated with poorer health were older age, poor income, no health insurance, and increasing number of chronic diseases. This analysis also showed how healthy ageing in later life is influenced by factors at the early, mid and later life stages, highlighting the importance of broad ranging policies across the age spectrum. It has demonstrated that in addition to standard risk factors relevant for western populations, factors specific to China such as diet, high smoking, internal migration, and use of traditional medications play an important role in the health and ageing of the population [30].

2.7 Successful Ageing Among Older People in China

An analysis of data from people aged ≥60 years in the China Health and Retirement Study, estimated that 13.2% of Chinese older people could be categorized as ageing successfully. These people had no major diseases, no disability, high cognitive functioning, high physical functioning, and active engagement with life. The percentages of older people with each of the individual indicators were 42% with no major diseases, 92% with no disability, 54% with high cognitive functioning, 70% with high physical functioning, and 46% with active engagement with life. People who had more education had better odds of successful ageing compared with those with less than primary school education, with this effect being stronger in women than men. Older people from a non-agricultural Hukou had an almost two-fold increase in the odds of successful ageing compared with people from an agricultural Hukou. Older people living in the central, northeast or western regions had lower odds of successful ageing relative to those living in the east coast region [34].

2.8 Dietary Transitions and Chronic Disease in China

Another large set of epidemiological data can be obtained from the Chinese Health and Nutrition Study. Evidence suggests few people met the Chinese dietary recommendations, with many having excess grains, oil, and salt. People living in medium and high urbanicity areas had significantly better dietary scores than those living in low urbanicity areas. Poorer diet quality was also associated with gender, with women having higher food scores, and education with higher food scores for those with greater levels of literacy [35].

Three dietary patterns were identified by factor analysis, labelled "Traditional Chinese", "Protein-rich", and "Starch-rich" dietary pattern. A protein-rich dietary pattern (high intake of milk, eggs, and soymilk) was associated with higher cognitive global scores and verbal memory scores, while the starch-rich dietary pattern (high intake of salted vegetable and legumes) was associated with lower scores. On longitudinal analysis, there was evidence that older people's diets were moving towards a modern dietary pattern (high intake of dairy, fruit, cakes, and fast food) [36].

Traditional and modern dietary patterns had clear associations with higher body mass index, weight, and waist circumference [36, 37]. The prevalence of general obesity was 9.5% and central obesity was 53.4%. Traditional dietary patterns (high intake of rice, pork, and vegetables) were inversely associated with general/central obesity; modern dietary patterns (high intake of fruit, fast food, and processed meat) were positively associated with general/central obesity [37]. Traditional dietary patterns were also inversely associated with hypertension [36]. Associations between modern dietary pattern and hypertension differed by urbanization, being inverse in areas of low urbanization, positive in medium urbanization, and no association in high urbanization. Dietary lead showed a significant positive association with hypertension that indicating high levels of concern on food contamination due to rapid industrialization and urbanization in China [38].

2.9 Policy Responses

The 2016–2020 five-year plan for China was informed by in-depth explorations and discussions of the implications of population ageing, and considering World Health Organization recommendations to improve the health and well-being of older populations. This plan included strengthening top level design, family planning policy, employment systems, care services, social security, health programmes, training systems, environmental support, and social participation [39]. The 2021–2025 plan extends these goals, and with additional attention to the long-term care needs of older people [40].

An analysis of Chinese ageing policies extracted from the Peking University Law database and websites of government departments shows how China's ageing policy has evolved over decades, moving from a focus on basic security to an emphasis on participation, integrated medical care, service quality, and human rights. Additionally, as time has gone by more and more government departments have become involved in the policy responses to population ageing and the needs of older people [41].

China has also been working on better integrated care, including the development of an internet-based medical information platform. The aim is to create an integrated, community-based social and health care system. These systems will complement strategies for chronic disease control and prevention, improved health services, and a larger health workforce [42].

2.10 Conclusion

Ageing is more than a biological process and is largely influenced by social and cultural circumstances. These circumstances exert their influence from the earliest stages of life, and throughout adult life. While there are some chances to "catch up" and change the course of ageing in later life, it is difficult to override the effects of life's foundations.

Cultural factors will also influence ageing, but these are not immutable. In China, for example, dramatic changes in lifestyle have accompanied rapid structural ageing. The effect has been a double whammy of an increasing proportion of older people, and increasing disease risk among those people. However, the Chinese governments have been conscientious to respond to these changes, recognizing that responding to ageing is not the sole purview of one department, nor indeed only concerning older people [42, 43].

References

1. Takács J, Nyakas C. The role of social factors in the successful ageing—systematic review. Dev Health Sci. 2022;4(1):11–20.
2. Marmot M. Social determinants of health inequalities. Lancet. 2005;365:1099–104.

3. Blane D, Higgs P, Hyde M, Wiggins RD. Life course influences on quality of life in early old age. Soc Sci Med. 2004;58:2171–9.
4. Schmitz LL, Zhao W, Ratliff SM, Goodwin J, Miao J, Lu Q, Guo X, Taylor KD, Ding J, Liu Y, Levine M. The socioeconomic gradient in epigenetic ageing clocks: evidence from the multi-ethnic study of atherosclerosis and the health and retirement study. Epigenetics. 2022;17(6):589–611.
5. Halleröd B, Gustafsson JE. A longitudinal analysis of the relationship between changes in socio-economic status and changes in health. Soc Sci Med. 2011;72:116–23.
6. Britton A, Shipley M, Singh-Manoux A, Marmot MG. Successful ageing: the contribution of early-life and midlife risk factors. J Am Geriatr Soc. 2008;56:1098–105.
7. Mishra G, Nitsch D, Black S, De Stavola B, Kuh D, Hardy R. A structured approach to modelling the effects of binary exposure variables over the life course. Int J Epidemiol. 2009;38:528–37.
8. Barker DJP. Fetal origins of coronary heart disease. BMJ. 1995;311(1):171–4.
9. Haapanen MJ, Perälä MM, Salonen MK, Kajantie E, Simonen M, Pohjolainen P, Eriksson JG, von Bonsdorff MB. Early life determinants of frailty in old age: the Helsinki birth cohort study. Age Ageing. 2018;47(4):569–75.
10. Wahrendorf M, Blane D, Bartley M, Dragano N, Siegrist J. Working conditions in mid-life and mental health in older ages. Adv Life Course Res. 2013;18(1):16–25.
11. Cullati S, Sieber S, van der Linden BW, Orsholits D, von Arx M, Boisgontier MP, Cheval B. Childhood socioeconomic disadvantage and health in the second half of life: The role of gender and welfare states in the life course of Europeans. In: Withstanding vulnerability throughout adult life: dynamics of stressors, resources, and reserves, vol. 14. Cham: Springer; 2023. p. 217–38.
12. Stringhini S, Zaninotto P, Kumari M, Kivimäki M, Lassale C, Batty GD. Socio-economic trajectories and cardiovascular disease mortality in older people: the English Longitudinal Study of Ageing. Int J Epidemiol. 2018;47(1):36–46.
13. Wildman JM, Moffatt S, Pearce M. Quality of life at the retirement transition: life course pathways in an early 'baby boom' birth cohort. Soc Sci Med. 2018;207:11–8.
14. Yang CY, Schorpp K, Boen C, Johnson M, Harris KM. Socioeconomic status and biological risks for health and illness across the life course. J Gerontol. 2020;75(3):613–24.
15. Kendig H, Loh V, O'Loughlin K, Byles J, Nazroo JY. Pathways to well-being in later life: socioeconomic and health determinants across the life course of Australian Baby Boomers. J Popul Ageing. 2016;9:49–67.
16. Burns RA, Loh V, Byles JE, Kendig HL. The impact of childhood parental quality on mental health outcomes in older adults. Aging Ment Health. 2018;22(6):819–25.
17. Yip APW, Nolte J, Loeckenhoff CE. Aging across the world: the interplay of demographic, economic, historical, and cultural factors. In: Drolet A, Yoon C, editors. The aging consumer: perspectives from psychology and marketing. 2nd ed. New York: Routledge; 2020. p. 259–78.
18. Bengtson V, Biblarz T, Clare E, Giarrusso R, Roberts R, Richlin-Klonsky J, Silverstein M. Intergenerational relationships and aging: families, cohorts, and social change. In: Clair JM, Allman R, editors. The gerontological prism: building interdisciplinary bridges. Boca Raton: CRC Press; 2018. p. 115–48.
19. Park L, Jacobs E. Cultural determinants of health and healthy ageing for older adults with limited-English proficiency. Innov Aging. 2018;2(Suppl 1):195.
20. Zeng L, Perry L, Xu X. Self-care behaviours and related cultural factors among Chinese immigrants with cardiovascular disease in western countries: an integrative review. J Clin Nurs. 2021;00:1–16.
21. Hung LW, Kempen GIJM, De Vries NK. Cross-cultural comparison between academic and lay views of healthy ageing: a literature review. Ageing Soc. 2010;30:8.
22. Chen X, Giles J, Yao Y, Yip W, Meng Q, Berkman L, Chen H, Chen X, Feng J, Feng Z, Glinskaya E. The path to healthy ageing in China: a Peking University–Lancet Commission. Lancet. 2022;400(10367):1967–2006.

23. Bedford O, Yeh K-H. The history and the future of the psychology of filial piety: the Chinese norms to contextualised personality construct. Front Psychol. 2019;10:100.
24. Chen T. Living arrangement preferences and realities for elderly Chinese: implications for subjective wellbeing. Ageing Soc. 2019;39(8):1557–81.
25. Kendig H, Gong CH, Yiengprugsawan V, Silverstein M, Nazroo J. Life course influences on later life health in China: childhood health exposure and socioeconomic mediators during adulthood. SSM Popul Health. 2017;3:795–802.
26. Yuan P, Xiang J, Borg M, Chen T, Lin X, Peng X, Zheng K. Analysis of lifetime death probability for major causes of death among residents in China. BMC Public Health. 2020;20:1–7.
27. Li R, Cheng X, Schwebel DC, et al. Disability-adjusted life years associated with population ageing in China, 1990–2017. BMC Geriatr. 2021;21:369.
28. Li Y, Teng DI, Shi X, Qin G, Qin Y, Quan H, Shi B, Sun H, Ba J, Chen B, Du J. Prevalence of diabetes recorded in mainland China using 2018 diagnostic criteria from the American Diabetes Association: national cross sectional study. BMJ. 2020;369:m997.
29. Hu X, Sun X, Li Y, Gu Y, Huang M, et al. Potential gains in health-adjusted life expectancy from reducing four main non-communicable diseases among Chinese elderly. BMC Geriatr. 2019;19:16.
30. Yiengprugsawan VS, Browning CJ. Non-communicable diseases and cognitive impairment: pathways and shared behavioral risk factors among older Chinese. Front Public Health. 2019;7:296.
31. Zhou M, Wang H, Zeng X, Yin P, Zhu J, Chen W, Li X, Wang L, Wang L, Liu Y, Liu J, Zhang M, Qi J, Yu S, Afshin A, Gakidou E, Glenn S, Krish VS, Miller-Petrie MK, Mountjoy-Venning WC, Mullany EC, Redford SB, Liu H, Naghavi M, Hay SI, Wang L, Murray CJL, Liang X. Mortality, morbidity, and risk factors in China and its provinces, 1990–2017: a systematic analysis for the Global Burden of Disease Study 2017. Lancet. 2019;394(10204):1145–58.
32. Wang M, Luo X, Xu S, Liu W, Ding F, Zhang X, Wang L, Liu J, Hu J, Wang W. Trends in smoking prevalence and implication for chronic diseases in China: serial national cross-sectional surveys from 2003 to 2013. Lancet Respir Med. 2019;7(1):35–45.
33. Biritwum RB, Minicuci N, Yawson AE, Theou O, Mensah GP, Naidoo N, Wu F, Guo Y, Zheng Y, Jiang Y, Maximova T, Kalula S, Arokiasamy P, Salinas-Rodríguez A, Manrique-Espinoza B, Snodgrass JJ, Sterner KN, Eick G, Liebert MA, Schrock J, Afshar S, Thiele E, Vollmer S, Harttgen K, Strulik H, Byles JE, Rockwood K, Mitnitski A, Chatterji S, Kowal P, WHO SAGE Collaboration. Prevalence of and factors associated with frailty and disability in older adults from China, Ghana, India, Mexico, Russia and South Africa. Maturitas. 2016;91:8–18.
34. Liu H, Byles JE, Xu X, Zhang M, Wu X, Hall JJ. Evaluation of successful aging among older people in China: Results from China health and retirement longitudinal study. Geriatr Gerontol Int. 2017;17:1183–90.
35. Xu X, Hall J, Byles J, Shi Z. Assessing dietary quality of older Chinese people using the Chinese Diet Balance Index (DBI). PLoS One. 2015;2015:10.
36. Xu X, Byles J, Shi Z, McElduff P, Hall J. Dietary pattern transitions, and the associations with BMI, waist circumference, weight and hypertension in a 7-year follow-up among the older Chinese population: a longitudinal study. BMC Public Health. 2016;16:743.
37. Xu X, Hall J, Byles J, Shi Z. Dietary pattern is associated with obesity in older people in China: data from China Health and Nutrition Survey (CHNS). Nutrients. 2015;7(9):8170–88.
38. Xu X, Byles JE, Shi Z, Hall JJ. Dietary patterns, dietary lead exposure and hypertension in the older Chinese population. Asia Pac J Clin Nutr. 2018;27(2):451–9.
39. The 13th Five-Year Plan for Economic And Social Development of The People's Republic Of China (2016–2020) https://en.ndrc.gov.cn/policies/202105/P020210527785800103339.pdf. Accessed 27 Jan 2023.

40. The State Council. The People's Republic of China. http://english.www.gov.cn/policies/latestreleases/202202/21/content_WS621357c5c6d09c94e48a5486.html. Accessed 30 Jan 2023.
41. Nan Y, Feng T, Hu Y, Qi X. Understanding aging policies in China: a bibliometric analysis of policy documents, 1978–2019. Int J Environ Res Public Health. 2020;17(16):5956. https://doi.org/10.3390/ijerph17165956. Published 2020 Aug 17.
42. Ageing and Health in China. https://www.who.int/china/health-topics/ageing.

Work and Retirement

3

Kate O'Loughlin, Vanessa Loh, and Martin Mackey

3.1 Introduction

Healthy ageing is shaped by experiences and outcomes related to working life and transition to and life in retirement. This chapter first provides an overview of older workers' participation in paid work and considers their key strengths and contributions, reasons for remaining employed, and work-related barriers frequently faced such as age discrimination, injury/illness, and carer responsibilities. A work ability framework is useful for understanding influences on older workers' continued workforce participation as it considers overall health and well-being (physical, psychological) and functional capacity and is included to gain an understanding of possible push/pull factors shaping decision-making around retirement. As discussed here, retirement is a major life transition and increasingly viewed as a process rather than one-off event. Pathways to retirement are identified such as moving to part-time or bridge employment, as well as the benefits of retirement planning and impact of voluntary versus involuntary retirement. The relationship of health status to retirement is considered with reference to differential occupational exposures, an increasingly casualised workforce and issues around work-life balance including differences in outcomes for men and women. Acknowledging the various factors influencing older workers' experiences, the chapter concludes with discussion of lifestyles in retirement that may be shaped by one's health status, age, gender, and level of financial security.

K. O'Loughlin (✉) · V. Loh · M. Mackey
The University of Sydney, Sydney, NSW, Australia
e-mail: kate.oloughlin@sydney.edu.au; vanessa.loh@sydney.edu.au; martin.mackey@sydney.edu.au

J. Byles (ed.), *What Matters for Healthy Ageing*, Topics in Geriatric Care, https://doi.org/10.1007/978-981-96-0462-3_3

3.2 Employment in Older Age

Employment patterns of older workers and possible pathways to retirement will vary significantly within and between countries. Sources of difference will be shaped by demographic factors such as gender, partnership status, race/ethnicity, socio-economic position, occupation, geographical location, health and/or disability status as well as the socio-political structures shaping policies and the social welfare and retirement income systems in place [1]. Evidence suggests that in the last 20–30 years older people (55–74 years) have extended their working lives; however, participation rates vary across countries [1–4]. Given this evidence and the fact that age-related compulsory retirement has been removed in many developed countries, early retirement still occurs [1]. For example, in 2018–2019 the average retirement age of all retirees in Australia was 55.4 years [5]. What is also evident in these changing patterns of employment is the gender differences with increasing participation of women in employment and declining participation rates for men; however, this does vary when considering full-time and part-time employment status [6, 7].

3.2.1 Socio-demographic Differences Contributing to Employment Status and Outcomes

The focus of much of the demographic and social gerontological research in population ageing has been on the post-Second World War baby boom cohorts generally defined as those born in the mid-to-late 1940s to mid-1960s. From a population ageing perspective, these baby boomers are the future older generation as they enter mid-to-later life and, in many ways, are redefining what ageing looks like compared with earlier generations [8–10]. While the baby boomers lived through periods of extensive social and economic change which shaped their attitudes, behaviours, expectations, and social networks, and continue to do so as they enter older age, they cannot be considered a homogeneous group as there is as much diversity with and between baby boom cohorts as there will be in any other generation, with different exposures and experiences across the life course shaped by factors such as socio-economic position, gender, partnership status, ethnicity, health status, and geographical location [8, 9, 11, 12]. They are now the focus of much public policy, especially around extended working lives and pension age eligibility, as governments attempt to manage public expenditure around a future heavily influenced by an ageing population [13–15]. In the Australian context, a public discourse on intergenerational inequity has emerged amid perceptions that the life prospects of younger age cohorts are declining when compared with the higher levels of home-ownership and retirement wealth attributed to many Australian baby boomers [8, 16].

Socio-economic position (SEP) can lead to inequalities which, in turn, pose risks to income security and health status at any life stage including older age and can be influenced by gender, ethnicity, partner status, health status, occupation, and geographical location [17, 18]. Using Australia as an example, labour force data indicate increased participation rates, particularly for women, and a high incidence of part-time work [19]. Women make up 38.4% of all full-time employees and 68.5% of all part-time employees [5, 20]. While baby boomer women led the way in taking up paid work, participation continues to be shaped by socio-cultural and economic factors associated with women's social roles including interrupted work histories and expectations of providing care at various life stages [21]. The gender pay gap and women's under-representation in senior management roles also present barriers to equal participation in paid employment [11, 20, 22].

A current global concern is the emergence of homelessness [11]. Using Australia as an example, there is concern over the increase in homelessness in all age groups and particularly for older women [23, 24]. A key risk factor identified for women as potentially leading to later life homelessness is financial difficulties [23]. As noted previously, women's employment histories can be shaped by periods of unemployment, underemployment, or extended periods in part-time work; additionally, in developed countries there is a high divorce rate, especially among baby boomers [25] with evidence to suggest financial stress as a particular outcome for women [26] thus influencing their income security across the life course and into older age. Also contributing to homelessness is the decline in the provision of affordable social housing and the introduction of market-driven systems of service provision including community and aged care [27].

Other key factors contributing to social and economic advantage/disadvantage and health status in older age are employment sector/industry, occupational status, and the availability of work opportunities [28, 29]. The exposures for those working in low-skilled, low-paid occupations, and/or non-standard and insecure forms of employment are significantly different to those in highly paid occupations and can lead to age-related inequalities that may start very early in life and accumulate over the life span [30–33]. Evidence from the UK indicates that four industries employ almost half (47%) of workers aged 50 and over; these are health, retail, education, and manufacturing [34]. These are industries often characterised by the gendered division of labour, requiring semi- to low-skilled workers, and with a high level of part-time and insecure engagement [35–37].

The Covid pandemic exposed the impact of occupational status and industry settings on workers whereby the impact both during and post-pandemic was highly influenced by one's skill set, education level, income, employment sector and, to some degree, gender, and age [6, 21, 35, 37–39]. While governments around the world provided financial support to businesses to retain employees and/or to those who became unemployed, this was generally for a limited time and benefited some more than others [6]. Industries with high levels of low-paid workers on non-standard contracts (variable hours of work, low hourly pay rate, no paid leave entitlements) such as hospitality, retail, tourism, and manufacturing had high levels of unemployment and underemployment resulting from extended periods of closure as working from home was not an option, while those in occupations with higher pay and paid leave entitlements (e.g. banking/finance, education, public service) had the flexibility to work from home and reduce their working hours through accessing leave entitlements [6, 35, 36, 40]. During lockdown periods, frontline workers in sectors such as health and social care were placed under considerable stress in Australia and elsewhere [40, 41]. Low-paid workers providing nursing assistance and personal care in aged and disability services, often older women from a non-English speaking background [42] were deemed 'essential workers'. However, the casual and insecure nature of their employment was exposed as many were 'second job holding' [41] in that they worked in multiple care sites for one employer or across a range of care sites for multiple employers. This work pattern was considered as spreading the virus both to clients and within their own families, but as workers employed on an hourly rate and without paid leave entitlements time away from work was not an option [37, 40].

3.2.2 Key Strengths and Contributions of Older Workers

While acknowledging the differential exposures outlined above, older workers are recognised for their contributions in the labour market [1, 31]. The positive attributes associated with older workers include their experience, knowledge and skills, reliability, stability, strong work ethic, mentoring capacity, and maintaining a positive attitude [31, 43]. These attributes of older workers have been acknowledged by governments in policy initiatives to support extended working lives and engage employers and industries in strategies to retain a more age-diverse workforce [1, 44].

The age one leaves paid work can be influenced by a range of individual and structural factors. While population ageing may be impacting on labour force participation, an older worker's reasons for remaining in paid work could be due to financial necessity, enjoyment and satisfaction in their work, and staying active and socially engaged [45]. However, an early exit might also occur due to illness, injury, or through redundancy [44].

3.2.3 Work-Related Barriers

While an extended working life is now an expectation for many older workers and encouraged by governments, there are several barriers that may prevent this being realised [1, 44]. Two potential barriers will be considered here: perceptions and experiences of ageism and age discrimination in workplaces and increased carer responsibilities, particularly for women, associated with increased life expectancy [11, 23].

Age discrimination: Age discrimination, at any age, is illegal in many countries; however, a major focus of ageing-related research has been around socio-cultural attitudes to ageing and the stereotypes of age and ageing depicted in all forms of media and also evident in workplaces [1, 46–48]. As mentioned previously, there are positive attributes associated with older workers, however from an employer and workplace perspective the focus is more likely to be on negative stereotypes very often related to perceptions of the older person as less capable of taking up new skills, resistant to change, inflexible in their attitudes and behaviours and, in the view of younger workers, often in the way of their own career progression [1, 49, 50]. One common assumption informing this view relates to their understanding and use of technology, often referred to as the 'digital divide', that separates the younger and older generations [51, 52] and there is evidence to suggest that some older workers are limited in the skills needed to operate in technology-rich environments [1, 53]. There is recognition by governments and advocacy groups of the impact of age discrimination in workplaces and attempts have been made to address the issue. For example, Australia's national government has provided financial incentives to employers to recruit mature age workers and established a Mature Age Hub to provide resources for both mature age workers (45+ years) and employers [54], while the Australian Human Rights Commission has developed an Older Workers Resource Hub [55].

In the workplace itself, negative attitudes towards older workers are often manifested in recruitment and retention practices and expressed in claims around low productivity and high labour costs [53]. However, the employability of older workers can be impacted by lack of training opportunities [1, 56], inflexible work practices pertaining to function and capacity [57, 58], and terminating employment based on ageist assumptions about their desire or need to remain in paid work [53]. An Australian study [49] based on a national survey sample (aged 18+ years) found that while Australia has legislation in place to address age discrimination particularly within employment, age discrimination was perceived as common, particularly among those in the main working age range of 35–49 (51%) and 50–64 years (48%), while participants across gender and age groups reported that compared to younger workers, older workers (55+ years) were more likely to be made redundant (77%), less likely to be promoted (67%), and more likely to have difficulty adapting to change (55%); however, the majority (70%) disagreed that older workers were less productive than younger workers.

The perpetuation of age discrimination in workplaces and employment practices has consequences in terms of opportunities, barriers, and fair treatment for all, but particularly for older workers and, in the longer term, for overall economic security. From a policy perspective, the question remains around what else can be done to address ageist attitudes and discriminatory behaviours generally, and specifically in the workplace. According to the OECD [11] what is needed to address the changing context of ageing and work at the individual, economic and societal level is a public policy agenda that supports the mobilisation, maintenance, and maximisation of a multigenerational workforce that recognises and values the contributions of workers of all ages and across gender, occupation, and industry.

Carer responsibilities: A consequence of government policy responses to the social and economic impact of population ageing is the increasing research focus on older working carers as they face pressures around remaining in and managing paid work alongside caring longer and more intensively for family members, often as a multigenerational carer for a spouse/partner, ageing parents, adult children with disabilities and grandchildren [48, 59–62]. While governments have recognised the role of carers through legislative and policy provisions, and globally many countries have policies in place to provide paid or unpaid carer leave and flexible work arrangements, available evidence suggests they are not always adequate if the care required is ongoing [59, 63]. In Australia working carers may be eligible for paid leave and have the right to request flexible work arrangements, but it depends on one's employment status. For example, those in full-time or part-time permanent employment have access to paid personal/carer's leave, paid compassionate leave, and flexible work arrangements; however, those in casual or insecure employment (hourly pay rate, variable hours) may take leave for carer responsibilities but it is unpaid [64, 65].

Common themes emerging from the international research literature on older working carers revolve around a range of social, economic, and health issues including the impact on workforce participation, health and well-being, and the nature and extent of care provided [66–69]. A major concern relates to income security and being expected to, or needing/wanting to remain in paid work, and dealing with the social, emotional, and financial impact of increased and enduring caring responsibilities for family members [49, 70, 71].

With population ageing men are taking up carer roles, particularly spousal/partner care; however, the available evidence suggests that working carers are more likely to be women, older, and with a lower employment rate than non-carers [5, 68, 72–74]. As previously mentioned, women have higher rates of casual and insecure employment than men [35, 40] and their participation in paid work is shaped by socio-cultural and economic factors associated with their social roles including interrupted work histories and providing care at various life stages [21, 72]. The demands and impact of caring on the health and well-being of the carer can be a major 'push' factor associated with moving to part-time work or leaving paid work [60, 63, 75].

An Australian study drawing on Carers NSW survey data (closed/open questions) at three time points (2014, 2016, 2018) found working carers were more likely to be women, a primary carer, aged 45–64 years, university educated, with 25% reporting having their own disability or long-term illness [59]. Participation in paid work changed across the survey periods with an increase in part-time and casual work evident in 2018 which may indicate an increase in carer responsibilities. Study participants indicated that paid work offered some respite from their caring role, but also reported it was stressful managing both, and they felt their situation hindered career development. With flexible work arrangements, the most commonly used options were carer's leave (paid, unpaid), flexible start-finish times, job sharing, and working from home although this varied across workplaces and remained a barrier for some due to the attitudes and lack of support of managers and co-workers [59].

In summary, older workers' participation in paid work has been increasing and will continue to grow; however, there needs to be recognition of the diversity and sources of difference shaping the experiences and outcomes for older workers based on a range of socio-demographic factors including gender, race/ethnicity, socio-economic position, occupation, geographical location, health status, and work-related barriers such as age discrimination and carer responsibilities. The next section draws on these factors within a work ability framework to understand the influences on older workers' continued workforce participation, particularly related to health and physical function and capacity. This framework considers a range of individual, organisational, and socio-structural factors shaping the experience of being in a worker role and has a particular relevance in the context of population ageing and expectations of extended working lives.

3.3 Promotion of Work Ability in Older Workers

Maintaining and promoting work ability over the life course is an important social objective. The 'work ability' construct concerns a worker's ongoing capacity to perform their work, including both an individual's personal resources and working conditions [76]. A holistic multidimensional work ability model, conceptualised as a 'house', was developed by researchers at the Finnish Institute of Occupational Health to conceptualise the construct (Fig. 3.1). The house consists of several 'floors' or levels comprising the resources of the individual worker (including health

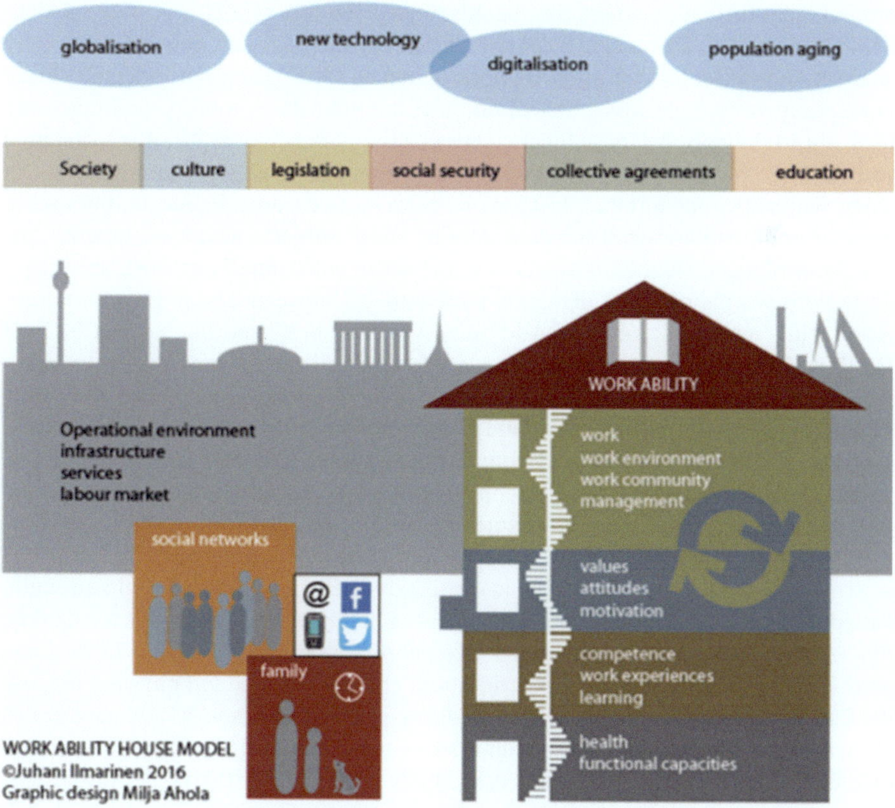

Fig. 3.1 The Work Ability House Model. (Source: Ilmarinen [77 , p. 3])

and functional capacities; knowledge and skills; values, attitudes, motivations), as well factors related to their work (working conditions, work content and demands, work community and organisation, supervision, and management). In addition, work ability can be influenced by the external factors such as organisations that support safe work, and by close family and community, and at a macro level by societal factors such as culture, legislation, social, health, and ageing policies [77].

Factors influencing the work ability of older workers have been extensively canvassed in numerous cohort studies over the last 30 years including [76, 78, 79]. Following a large population-based Finnish study, Gould et al. [76] reported that work ability declined with increasing age in both men and women but was higher in employed persons compared with those unemployed and the total population. Work ability was also limited in those less educated, those with lower physical and social functioning, job insecurity, in part-time and lower skilled work, and for those with greater job dissatisfaction.

More recently the Health and Employment After 50 (HEAF) prospective cohort study was conducted among a population of 8134 adults aged 50–64 years, recruited from 24 English GP practices [76]. This research group investigated whether the 'frailty' phenotype (which predicts adverse events in older age) is associated with employment difficulties including health-related job loss (HRJL), prolonged sickness absence (>20 days vs. less, past 12 months), having to cut down substantially at work and difficulty coping with work demands [80]. Using the (adapted) Fried et al. criteria of weight loss, exhaustion, grip strength, slow mobility, and inactivity [81], approximately 4% of subjects were classed at baseline as 'frail' (3–5 items) and 32% as 'pre-frail' (1–2 items). Three-quarters of 'frail' subjects were not in work, while 60% had left their last job on health grounds, an outcome 30 times more likely in frail than non-frail subjects. Among 'frail' subjects who were in work, the risk for prolonged sickness absence, cutting down substantially at work and struggling with work's physical demands increased by between 11- and 17-fold compared with 'non-frail' subjects. Additionally, it was predicted that almost 52% of HRJL and 37% of extended sick leave would be eliminated if any one frailty criterion present could be prevented. Associations were strongest for those with slow reported walking speed [80]. At 4- and 5- year follow-up, slower walking speed was associated with lower socio-economic status, lower physical activity, obesity, greater job dissatisfaction and not coping at work physically and/or mentally, and the adjusted risk of HRJL was 2–3 times greater for men and women with very slow walking speed compared to those with normal or faster walking speed [82, 83].

It is well documented that physical capacity (aerobic fitness, muscle strength, and joint flexibility) declines with age, and after 50 years the decline is more marked [84]. Aerobic fitness declines about 1–2% per year after the age of 20–25 [85] due predominately to physiological deterioration, chronic disease, and physical inactivity. Further, muscle mass reduces by 0.3–0.5% per year after age 30 and accelerates after age 60 due to reduced number and size of muscle fibres [86]. The determinants of muscle function also include gender, body mass index (BMI), comorbidities, mood, cognitive function, diet, and leisure-time physical activity (LTPA) [82]. It is well known that LTPA is beneficial in promoting health and wellness, reducing obesity, improving cardiovascular fitness, and reducing falls and fractures. However, a lifetime of occupational physical workload does not have similar training effects on individual physical work capacity as does aerobic physical exercise. Indeed, physical work capacity declines with age in physical occupations as much, or even more, than in mentally demanding occupations [87–89]. A 2-year follow-up study of HEAF study participants also found that older workers employed as road transport drivers or in vehicle trades (men), or as teaching/education and nursing/midwifery professionals or in caring personal services (women), were more frequently among those exiting work for health-related versus non-health-related reasons [90]. Further, the main socio-demographic and lifestyle risk factors for HRJL for those exiting employment were 'struggling financially' (men and women); low physical activity (men); being overweight or obese, and current smoking (women). Those older workers with poor self-perceived health status were 2–3 times at greater risk of HRJL, and men with high physical occupational workloads were at a 160% greater risk for HRJL during this follow-up period [91].

In a study investigating factors influencing the dimensions of work ability in underground coal workers Mackey et al. [92] found older workers perceived they had significantly less training opportunities, more discrimination and less respect, and lower career support compared to younger workers. In addition, older workers had more injuries and diseases, poorer work/life balance, and lower overall work ability.

Health and job satisfaction are known to be key independent determinants of the ability to work to older ages [93, 94]. However, it also appears that these important factors may interact synergistically on health-related job loss (HRJL) in older workers. D'Angelo et al. [95] reported that among the 5143 HEAF study participants who were ever in work in the study period, 5.7% and 14.3% of men, in good and poor self-rated health, respectively, reported job dissatisfaction, while among women these percentages were 4.6 and 12.9. In addition, men in good health dissatisfied with their job had a sixfold (HR = 6.4; 95% CI 3.3–12.4) increased risk of HRJL compared with men satisfied with their job (a significant multiplicative interaction) [95].

The promotion of work ability over the life course involves directing strategies to address deficits in one or more of these multidimensional factors with the aim of promoting good work ability and health, good work quality and productivity, good quality of life and well-being, and active and meaningful retirement [96]. The work ability promotion concept is based on four different actions: (i) adjustments needed in the physical work environment, (ii) adjustments needed in the psychosocial work environment, (iii) health and lifestyle promotion, and (iv) updating professional skills (Fig. 3.2) [97].

Various health and lifestyle promotion strategies have been tested among older workers in numerous workplace settings. For example, in underground coal workers exposed to a 16-week health and wellness promotion programme, being more physically active in leisure time was associated with less injury and disease, less fatigue, better psychological health, and better overall self-rated work ability [92]. Similarly, significant improvements in physical activity, health status, and work ability were

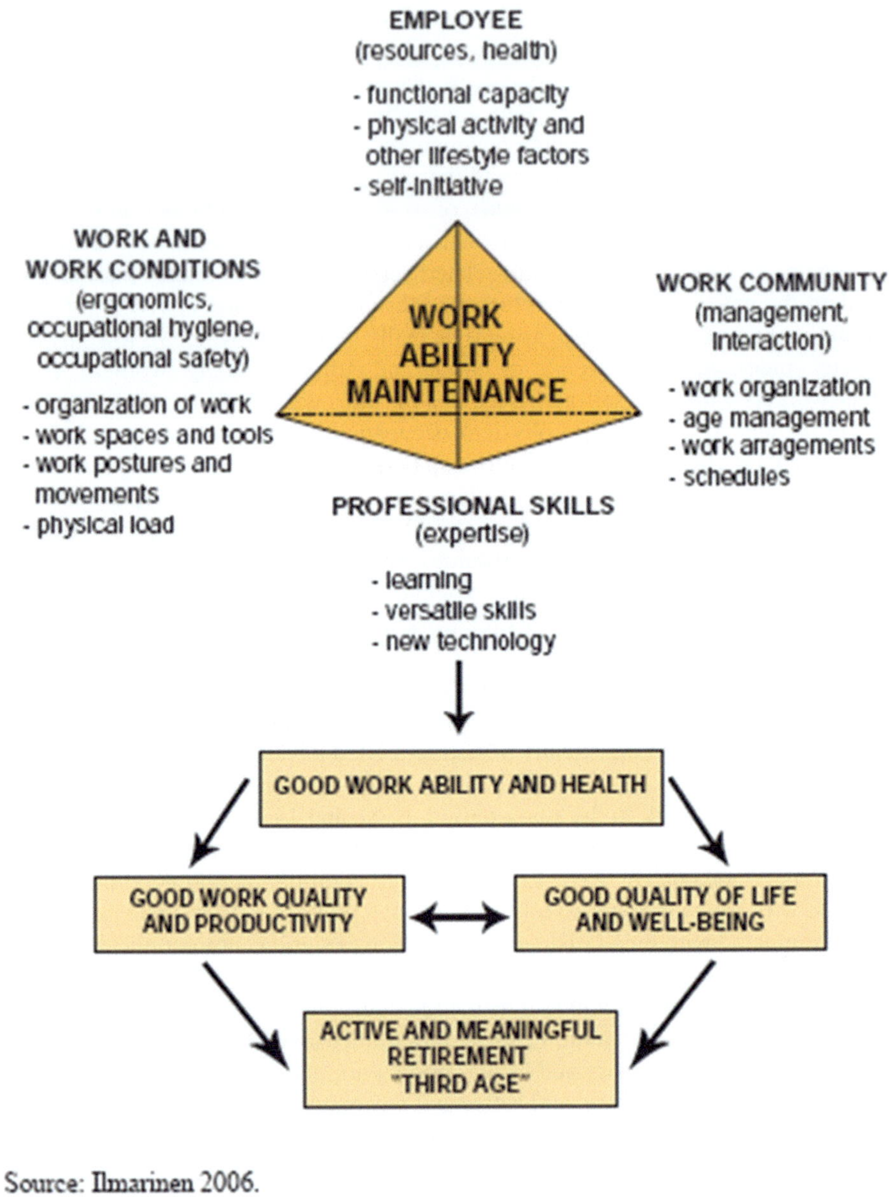

Fig. 3.2 Promotion of work ability in older workers. (Source: Ilamarinen (2006) cited in Gould et al. [69, p. 21])

also found by a randomised controlled study investigating a flexible, individually targeted worksite-based walking intervention to fit around working life, using behaviour change principles, in sedentary university employees [98, 99].

A recent systematic review [100] analysed whether workplace interventions positively impact work ability. The authors reviewed 17 randomised control trials [45] (comprising 22 articles) comprising multilevel interventions (N = 5) including changes to work arrangements and liaisons with supervisors, and individual-focused interventions (N = 12) involving behaviour change or exercise programmes. The meta-analysis showed a small positive significant effect [overall pooled mean 0.12, 95% CI 0.03–0.21], suggesting that workplace interventions might improve work ability. However, the quality of the evidence base was only moderate, precluding any firm conclusion [100]. Several suggestions have been posited to improve the effectiveness of interventions [77]. Organisations should give timelier prioritisation to addressing identified risks for poor work ability among their employees. Second, efforts should be made to increase participation rates of workers in interventions, whether these are focussed on health and lifestyle promotion or updating professional skills. Third, an outcome sensitive enough to measure change in work ability following intervention is crucial. The gold standard Work Ability Index (WAI) was originally developed for measuring work ability in research and industry studies from the 1980s [97]. In practice, however, the WAI is found to be a very challenging outcome to measure change for interventions, especially among older workers who easily face the age-related changes in personal resources and health [77], and thus broader measurements of work ability are necessary [101].

In summary, when the balance between work, human resources, and the environment creates positive effects on values, attitudes, and motivation of staff, both the work ability and workplace well-being will benefit workers, and especially older workers for an active and meaningful transition to retirement. The next section expands on the push/pull factors shaping retirement decision-making [102] particularly as they relate to health status and draws on the individual, socio-structural, financial, and organisational factors outlined above in considering the retirement process.

3.4 Retirement and Health in Retirement

The relationship between health and retirement is a complex one and the direction and nature of the relationship can vary greatly between individuals [103]. For example, changes in health may encourage some individuals to retire earlier than planned, while others may decide to remain in paid work to keep mentally active, to retain access to work benefits such as healthcare and insurance, or for other reasons unrelated to their health. Similarly, retirement can impact health in different ways, with some individuals experiencing health declines, some experiencing health improvements, and others experiencing stable health in retirement [104].

According to the Constitution of the World Health Organization [105], health may be broadly defined as 'a state of complete physical, mental and social well-being and not merely the absence of disease or infirmity'. Although the experience of each type of well-being is likely to vary significantly between individuals, the relationship between health and retirement may also vary as a function of the time spent in retirement [106]. Other factors that may significantly influence an individual's health in retirement include their control over the retirement decision (voluntary or involuntary), their retirement timing (early, on-time, or late), their social networks (e.g. having a partner, spouse, or close family or friends to catch up with), their socio-economic position (education and financial position), and paid work conditions (e.g. being engaged in flexible, meaningful work and working for socioemotional reasons vs financial reasons). The significant body of research on retirement outcomes suggest that the direction and magnitude of effects of retirement on various health outcomes are likely to depend in part on the pre-retirement and concurrent circumstances, including one's pre-retirement health, work conditions and work status, and access to financial as well as social supports [107, 108].

In their systematic review on the health effects of working past age 64, Baxter et al. [109] found positive or neutral effects on physical health and overall health status, but mixed effects on mental health. The positive effects of work on health are most likely to be experienced by males, those working part-time or reducing to part-time work, while negative effects are most likely to be experienced by those working in low quality, high demand, or low reward jobs. Baxter et al. [109] note that these differential effects of health in retirement raise questions about the potential for widening health and social inequalities between those who can choose how and when to retire from paid work, compared to those who have little choice in the decision of whether to retire, reduce their work hours, or continue working.

In another recent systematic review and meta-analysis on the relationship between work and mortality, Sewdas et al. [110] found that while early retirement was not associated with mortality risk, on-time retirement was. Specifically, they found that in studies that did not adjust for prior health, on-time retirement was significantly associated with a higher mortality risk compared to working past retirement. However, in the subgroup of studies that adjusted for prior health, on-time retirement was not significantly associated with mortality risk, highlighting the importance of considering the potential selection effects of health prior to retirement.

Analysing longitudinal panel data from 2956 workers aged 51–62 years of age in the 1992 wave of the US Health and Retirement Study (HRS), who had retired by 2010, Wu et al. [111] classed retirees as either healthy or unhealthy, depending on whether they rated poor health as important or not for retirement. Although the average retirement age was similar for both the healthy (M = 64.9, SD = 3.8) and unhealthy retiree subgroups (M = 64.3, SD = 4.1), unhealthy retirees had an 84% higher mortality risk than healthy retirees. When analysing each subgroup separately, they found that retiring later was related to lower all-cause mortality risk in both subgroups, suggesting that working longer may have positive health benefits as reflected in the lower mortality risk, regardless of whether or not poor health was a reason for retirement.

A larger study by Gorry et al. [106] analysing data from 10,535 individuals, including both the original 1992 and later HRS cohorts (up to 2014), found that while retirement was significantly associated with an increase in the number of health conditions, there was no significant change in self-reported overall health or mental health following retirement. Interestingly, after correcting for potential selection effects into retirement such as participants' age eligibility for government and employer-sponsored pensions, Gorry et al. [106] found that retirement was significantly associated with improvements in self-reported health, mental health, life satisfaction, and functional limitations, with many of these health-related improvements emerging after the first 4 years of retirement.

These mixed and often contradictory findings highlight some of the inherent complexities in trying to investigate and tease apart the effects of retirement on health, without also considering the potential selection effects of prior health on the decision to retire [103]. While poor health does not always lead to retirement, and retirement is often driven by reasons unrelated to health [112], changes in health are more likely to impact retirement decisions than changes in income or wealth, and poor health is consistently found to be a significant predictor of early and on-time retirement [107].

A recent study by Han [112] tries to better account for the potentially bidirectional relationship between retirement and health, using data from 9347 HRS participants aged 51 or older (between 1998 and 2016) to investigate changes in health following retirement transitions that were driven either by poor health or by reasons unrelated to health. Over the 18-year data collection period, around 62% of participants transitioned to full retirement, with only about a third of retirements due to poor health. Compared to participants who continued working, those who retired due to non-health reasons reported better self-rated health and mental health, while those who retired due to health reasons reported poorer self-rated health and mental health. Even after adjusting for significant pre-retirement health differences, only participants who retired due to poor health showed significant changes in self-rated health and mental health, with both health outcomes worsening following retirement. In contrast, those who retired for non-health reasons, showed no significant changes in health. These findings further highlight the need for future research to look more closely at health outcomes for different retiree subgroups, and in particular, those for whom retirement may have been due to poor health or other factors that potentially undermine an individual's sense of choice and control in relation to the timing and nature of their retirement. As noted by Han [112], two important areas for future research are identifying health-promoting factors that can benefit mature workers who have poor health and identifying ways to promote the health and well-being of individuals who retire due to poor health in addition to those who retire for reasons unrelated to their health.

While the emerging body of research on health in retirement continues to yield some mixed results, it is clear that the relationship between health and retirement is complex. For some individuals, health will significantly influence their decision to retire, while for others it will play less of a defining role. Similarly, for some individuals, retiring from paid work may accelerate health declines, while for others; it may result in health gains or little impact on health, above and beyond retirement-independent, age-related changes. Essentially, a challenge for future research will be to better acknowledge and address the great diversity that exists between individuals in terms of their work and retirement experiences, the many potential effects of health and non-health factors on retirement, and the many potential effects of retirement on an individual's physical, mental, and social health and well-being.

3.5 Lifestyle in Retirement

In considering retirement lifestyles, the research literature conceptualises it in four ways: continuing a pre-retirement lifestyle; starting afresh; a form of imposed disruption; and transitioning to old age [113]. The social and economic circumstances of the post-Second World War baby boomer cohorts may mean many remain in some form of paid employment for longer than previous generations and, as such, delay moving to a near-total leisure lifestyle in retirement [9]. However, as outlined above the timing of retirement and level of activity and social engagement in retirement may be shaped by the interplay between one's physical and mental health status and levels of financial security.

Across the life course, social engagement is widely regarded as an important determinant of health and well-being, but particularly so into late adulthood and the retirement life stage [114, 115]. Positive discourses such as 'successful ageing' and 'productive ageing' are often applied to convey expectations for individuals to maintain independence, health, and well-being by minimising disease and disability and remaining physically active and socially engaged [32, 116]. This emphasis on physical health, including disease and disability age-related profiles, is often central in service delivery models related to retirement and older age [117]; however, others are critical of this one-dimensional focus and call for models that aim to improve older adults' overall health through social engagement and participation [118]. Such an approach will assist in maintaining social and cultural connections within the community and result in greater benefits for both the individual and wider society. The commonly applied indicators of social engagement and participation include involvement in giving/receiving social support; satisfaction derived from the support received from others; presence of a confidant; social activities (e.g. membership of clubs, religious affiliation, volunteering, family activities); and use of time (e.g. hours spent outside the home) [115].

3.6 Conclusion

This chapter provided an overview of older workers' participation in paid work generally and specifically within the context of population ageing, increased life expectancy, and the expectation of extended working lives. While identifying their strengths and contributions, recognition of the diversity and sources of difference that shape the experiences and outcomes for older workers were also addressed; these included gender, partnership status, race/ethnicity, socio-economic position, occupation, geographical location, health status, work-related barriers such as age discrimination, injury/illness, and carer responsibilities, and the socio-political structures shaping policies relevant to retirement income systems.

A work ability framework was applied to gain an understanding of possible push/pull factors shaping decision-making around retirement particularly as they relate to overall health and well-being (physical, psychological), functional capacity, and the workplace environment. While retirement remains a major life transition it is increasingly viewed as a process rather than one-off event, thus the various pathways to retirement were identified and discussed along with the scope and benefits of retirement planning and impact of voluntary versus involuntary retirement. The relationship of health status to retirement was considered within the context of differential occupational exposures, an increasingly insecure workforce, and issues around work-life balance including differences in outcomes for men and women that impact on both working and retirement lifestyles.

References

1. OECD. Working better with age, ageing and employment policies. Paris: OECD Publishing; 2019. https://doi.org/10.1787/c4d4f66a-en.
2. Geppert C, Guillemette Y, Morgavi H, Turner D. Labour supply of older people in advanced economies: the impact of changes to statutory retirement ages; 2019.
3. Key Policies to promote working lives. Country Note 2007–2017. OECD; 2018. https://www.oecd.org/els/emp/Poland%20Key%20policies_Final.pdf.
4. OECD. Retaining talent at all ages, ageing and employment policies. Paris: OECD Publishing; 2023. https://doi.org/10.1787/00dbdd06-en.
5. Australian Bureau of Statistics. Retirement and Retirement Intentions, AustraliaRetiree statistics and the retirement plans of people aged 45 years and over; 2020. https://www.abs.gov.au/statistics/labour/employment-and-unemployment/retirement-and-retirement-intentions-australia/latest-release. Accessed 1 Aug 2022.
6. OECD. OECD employment outlook 2021: navigating the COVID-19 crisis and recovery. Paris: OECD Publishing; 2021.
7. Gustafsson L. Australian labour force participation: historical trends and future prospects. Treasury Working Paper 2021–2. Canberra: Commonwealth of Australia; 2021.
8. O'Loughlin K, Hussain R, Kendig H. Attitudes towards Australia's baby boomers and intergenerational equity. Sociol Rev. 2021;69(4):792–811.
9. O'Loughlin K, Barrie H, Kendig H. Australia's baby boomers as the future older generation. In: Klassen T, editor. Ageing in Asia-Pacific: interdisciplinary and comparative perspectives. London: Routledge; 2018.
10. Leach R, Phillipson C, Biggs S, Money A. Baby boomers, consumption and social change: the bridging generation? Int Rev Sociol. 2013;23(1):104–22.
11. OECD. Promoting an age-inclusive workforce: living, learning and earning longer. Paris: OECD Publishing; 2020.
12. Tavener M, Byles J, Loxton D. Expert perceptions of the popular baby boomer image. Aust J Ageing. 2014;33(4):E31–5.
13. OECD. Pensions at a glance 2023: OECD and G20 Indicators. Paris: OECD Publishing; 2023. https://doi.org/10.1787/678055dd-en.
14. Cannon L, Kendig H. 'Millennials': perceived generational opportunities and intergenerational conflict in Australia. Australas J Ageing. 2018;37(4). Retrieved 3 29, 2023, from https://onlinelibrary.wiley.com/doi/full/10.1111/ajag.12566.
15. Kohli M, Arza C. The political economy of pension reform in Europe. In: Binstock R, George L, editors. Handbook of ageing and the social sciences. 7th ed. Cambridge, MA: Academic Press; 2011. p. 251–664.
16. Productivity Commission. Why did young people's incomes decline? Commission research paper. Productivity Commission: Canberra; 2020.
17. Stopforth S, Kapadia D, Nazroo J, Becares L. Ethnic inequalities in health in later life, 1993–2017: the persistence of health disadvantage over more than two decades. Ageing Soc. 2021;31(3):273–91.
18. Nazroo J. Class and health inequality in later life: patterns, mechanisms and implications for policy. Int J Environ Res Pub Health. 2017;14(12):1533.

19. Sila U, Dugain V. Income, wealth and earnings inequality in Australia: Evidence from the HILDA survey. OECD Economics Department Working Papers No. 1538. Paris: OECD Publishing; 2019.
20. Workplace Gender Equality. Gender equality workplace statistics at a glance 2022. Canberra: Australian Government; 2022.
21. Foley M, Cooper R. Workplace gender equality in the post-pandemic era: where to next? J Ind Relat. 2021;63(4):463–76.
22. Austen S, Mavisakalyan A. Gender gaps in long-term earnings and retirement wealth: The effects of education and parenthood. J Ind Relat. 2018;60(4):492–516.
23. Australian Human Rights Commission. Older women's risk of homelessness: background paper. Sydney: AHRC; 2019.
24. Australian Association of Gerontology. Background paper: older women experiencing, or at risk of, homelessness. Melbourne: Australian Association of Gerontology; 2018.
25. Crowley JE. Gray divorce: explaining midlife marital splits. J Women Aging. 2019;31(1):49–72.
26. Lichtenstein B, Lucke J, Loxton D. Women and divorce: financial coping from midlife to older age. J Women Aging. 2022;34(3):323–40.
27. Fine M, Davidson B. The marketization of care: global challenges and national responses in Australia. Curr Sociol Monogr. 2018;66(4):503–16.
28. Schram JL, Solovieva S, Leinonen T, Viikari-Juntura E, Burdorf A, Robroek SJ. The influence of occupational class and physical workload on working life expectancy among older employees. Scand J Work Environ Health. 2021;47(1):5–14.
29. Ravesteijn B, van Kippersluis H, van Doorslaer E. The contribution of occupation to health inequality. Res Econ Inequal. 2013;21:311–32.
30. Lain D, Phillipson C. Extended work lives and the rediscovery of the 'disadvantaged' older worker. Generations. 2019;43(3):71–7.
31. Noone J, Bohle P. Enhancing the health and employment participation of older workers. In: O'Loughlin K, Browning C, Kendig H, editors. Ageing in Australia: challenges and opportunities. New York: Springer; 2017. p. 127–46.
32. Kendig H, Loh V, O'Loughlin K, Byles J, Nazroo JY. Pathways to well-being in later life: socioeconomic and health determinants across the life course of Australian baby boomers. J Popul Ageing. 2016;9:49–67.
33. Dannefer D, Settersten R. The study of the life course: implications for social gerontology. In: Dannefer D, Phillipson C, editors. The SAGE handbook of social gerontology. London: Sage; 2010. p. 3–19.
34. Boys J. Megatrends: ageing gracefully: the opportunities of an older workforce. London: CIPD; 2019.
35. OECD. OECD employment outlook 2022: building back more inclusive labour markets. Paris: OECD Publishing; 2022.
36. Gilfillan G. Recent and long-term trends in the use of casual employment. Parliamentary Library: Canberra; 2021.
37. O'Neil M. The Australian industrial system in the era of COVID-19. J Ind Relat. 2021;63(3):422–31. https://doi.org/10.1177/00221856211012827.
38. Ksinan Jiskrova G, Bobák M, Pikhart H, Ksinan AJ. Job loss and lower healthcare utilisation due to COVID-19 among older adults across 27 European countries. J Epidemiol Community Health. 2021;75(11):1078–83.
39. Marmot M, Allen J. COVID-19: exposing and amplifying inequalities. J Epidemiol Community Health. 2020;74:681–2.
40. Stanford J. Shock troops of the pandemic: casual and insecure work in COVID and beyond. Canberra: Centre for Future Work, The Australia Institute. Canberra; 2021.
41. Baughman RA, Stanley B, Smith KE. Second job holding among direct care workers and nurses: implications for COVID-19 transmission in long-term care. Med Care Res Rev. 2022;79(1):151–60.

42. Charlesworth S, Isherwood L. Migrant aged-care workers in Australia: do they have poorer-quality jobs than their locally-born counterparts? Ageing Soc. 2021;41(12):2702–22.
43. Heisler W, Bandow D. Retaining and engaging older workers: a solution to worker shortages in the U.S. Bus Horiz. 2018;61(3):421–30.
44. Edgell V, Maclean G, Raeside R, Chen T. Age management in the workplace: manager and older worker accounts of policy and practice. Ageing Soc. 2020;40(4):784–804.
45. Loh V, Hamilton M, Baird M, Zettna N, Constantin A, Andrei DM, Petery GA, Parker SK. Money matters, but what else? Mature worker motives and the importance of gender, age, socioeconomic status and age-inclusive HR practices. Aust J Manag. 2024;49(4):790–811. https://doi.org/10.1177/03128962231176322.
46. World Health Organization. Global report on ageism. Geneva: WHO; 2021.
47. Loos E, Ivan L. Visual ageism in the media. In: Ayalon L, Tesch-Roemer C, editors. Contemporary aspects on ageism. Berlin: Springer; 2018. p. 163–76.
48. O'Loughlin K, Loh V, Kendig H. Carer characteristics and health, wellbeing and employment outcomes of older Australian baby boomers. J Cross Cult Gerontol. 2017;32(3):339–56.
49. O'Loughlin K, Kendig H, Hussain R, Cannon L. Age discrimination in the workplace: The more things change…. Australas J Ageing. 2017;36(2):98–101.
50. Clarke LH, Korotchenko A. 'I know it exists ... But I haven't experienced it personally': older Canadian men's perceptions of ageism as a distant social problem. Ageing Soc. 2016;1(8):1–17. 2015
51. Lovarini M, O'Loughlin K, Clemson L. Older adults and digital technologies. In: Sttrill-Smith A, Fullwood C, Keep M, Kuss D, editors. The Oxford handbook of cyberpsychology. 2nd ed. Oxford: Oxford University; 2019.
52. Neves BB, Waycott J, Malta S. Old and afraid of new communication technologies? Reconceptualising and contesting the 'age-based digital divide'. J Sociol. 2018;54(2):236–48.
53. Axelrad H, James JB. Employers' attitudes toward older-worker job seekers: a comprehensive review with recommendations for action. In: Antoniou A-S, Burke RJ, Cooper SC, editors. The aging workforce handbook. Bingley: Emerald Group Publishing Limited; 2016. p. 489–512.
54. Department of Employment and Workplace Relations. Mature age hub: a workforce Australia program [Internet]. Canberra: Department of Employment and Workplace relations; 2022. Available from: https://www.dewr.gov.au/mature-age-hub.
55. Australian Human Rights Commission. Older Workers Resource Hub [Internet]. Sydney: AHRC; 2022. [cited 2022 September 1]. Available from: https://humanrights.gov.au/olderworkers.
56. Loh V, Baird M. Supporting retirement pathways for older workers. In: Baird M, Hamilton M, Williams A, editors. The multigenerational workforce: managing age and gender at work; 2024. p. 209–36.
57. Seeberg KGV, Skovlund SV, Bláfoss R, Thomassen K, Malchow-Møller L, Sundstrup E, Andersen LL. The interplay between multimorbidity, physical work demands and work ability: cross-sectional study among 12,879 senior workers. Int J Environ Res Pub Health. 2022;19:5023.
58. Loh V, O'Loughlin K, Zettna N. Job design for age-inclusive workplaces. In: Baird M, Hamilton M, Williams A, editors. The multigenerational workforce: managing age and gender at work; 2024. p. 157–80.
59. O'Loughlin K, Triandafilidis Z, Rudd-Lam S. How flexible is flexible? Australia's flexible work policies to support working carers. Paper presented in Symposium Innovation for sustainable care: international perspectives from industry and practice, Transforming care conference, Copenhagen, 24–26 June 2019.
60. Phillips J, O'Loughlin K. Older workers and caregiving in a global context. J Cross Cult Gerontol. 2017;32:283–9. https://doi.org/10.1007/s10823-017-9328-2. Hill et al.
61. Loretto W, Vickerstaff S. Gender, age and flexible working in later life. Work Employ Soc. 2015;29(2):1–17.

62. Hamilton M, Baird M, Zettna N. Accommodating care across the life course. In: Baird M, Hamilton M, Williams A, editors. The multigenerational workforce: managing age and gender at work; 2024. p. 123–56.
63. Austin A, Heyes J. Supporting working carers: how employers and employees can benefit. Report prepared in collaboration with sustainable care: connecting people and systems programme and CIPD. Sheffield: The University of Sheffield; 2020.
64. Fair Work Commission. General protections benchbook. Canberra: Commonwealth of Australia; 2022.
65. O'Loughlin K, Williams A. Carer leave policies in Australia. In: Hamblin K, Heyes J, Fast J, editors. Combining work and care: carer leave and related employment policies in international context. Bristol UK: Bristol University Press; 2024. https://bristoluniversitypress.co.uk/combining-work-and-care.
66. Temple J, Dow B, Baird M. Special working arrangements to allow for care responsibilities in Australia: availability, usage and barriers. Aust Popul Stud. 2019;3(1):13–29.
67. Bainbridge HTJ, Broady TR, Fong MM. Individualized funding: How disability service policy can assist in maintaining caregiver employment. J Bus Manag. 2016;22(1):23–38.
68. Yeandle S, Buckner L. Older workers and care-giving in England: The policy context for older workers' employment patterns. J Cross Cult Gerontol. 2017;32(3):303–21. https://doi.org/10.1007/s10823-017-9332-6.
69. Alpass F, Szabo A, Allen J, Stephens C. Health effects of informal caring in New Zealand: longitudinal findings from the Health, Work and Retirement study. Int J Care Caring. 2017;1(3):309–29.
70. Duncan K, Shooshtari S, Kerstin R, Fast J, Han J. The cost of caring: out-of-pocket expenditures and financial hardship among Canadian carers. Int J Care Caring. 2020;4(2):141–66.
71. Hamilton and Jenkins 2015, Grandparent childcare and labour market Participation in Australia; 2015.
72. European Institute for Gender Equality. Gender inequalities in care and consequences for the labour market. Luxembourg: Publications Office of the European Union; 2021.
73. Charmes J. The unpaid care work and the labour market. An analysis of time use data based on the latest world compilation of time-use surveys. Geneva: International Labour Office; 2019.
74. Lei L, Leggett AN, Maust DT. A national profile of sandwich generation caregivers providing care to both older adults and children. J Am Geriatr Soc. 2023;71(3):799–809. https://doi.org/10.1111/jgs.18138.
75. Loh and Kendig, Kendig H. Australian developments in ageing: issues and history. In: O'Loughlin K, Browning C, Kendig H, editors. Ageing in Australia: challenges and opportunities. Cham: Springer; 2017. p. 13–27.
76. Gould R, Ilmarinen J, Jarvisalo J, Koskinen, editors. Dimension of work ability: results of the Health 2000 Survey. EU: Finnish Centre of Pensions (ETK), The Social Insurance Institution (KELA), National Public Health Institute (KTL), Finnish Institute of Occupational Health (FIOH), Helsinki, Finland; 2008.
77. Ilmarinen J. From work ability research to implementation Int. J Environ Res Public Health. 2019;16:2882.
78. Ilmarinen J, Tuomi K, Klockars M. Changes in the work ability of active employees over an 11-year period. Scand J Work Environ Health. 1997;23:49–57.
79. Palmer KT, Walker-Bone K, Harris EC, Linaker C, D'Angelo S, Sayer AA, Gale CR, Evandrou M, Van Staa T, Cooper C, Coggon D. Health and Employment after Fifty (HEAF): a new prospective cohort study. BMC Public Health. 2015;15(1):1–3.
80. Palmer KT, D'Angelo S, Harris EC, Linaker C, Gale CR, Evandrou M, Syddall H, van Staa T, Cooper C, Aihie Sayer A, Coggon D, Walker-Bone K. Frailty, prefrailty and employment outcomes in Health and Employment After Fifty (HEAF) Study. Occup Environ Med. 2017 Jul;74(7):476–82.
81. Fried LP, Tangen CM, Walston J, Newman AB, Hirsch C, Gottdiener J, Seeman T, Tracy R, Kop WJ, Burke G, McBurnie MA. Cardiovascular health study collaborative research group. Frailty in older adults: evidence for a phenotype. J Gerontol A Biol Sci Med Sci. 2001;56:M146–56.

82. Walker-Bone. Maximizing function and work ability throughout the life course. In: Proceedings workplace injury prevention and recovery, virtual THRIVE conference, Australian Physiotherapy Association, 11 May 2022; 2022.
83. Syddall HE, Ntani G, Bevilacqua G, et al. Slow walking speed and healthrelated exit from employment among older workers over 5 years of follow-up: evidence from the Health and Employment After Fifty (HEAF) cohort study. BMJ Open. 2024;14:e081509. https://doi.org/10.1136/bmjopen-2023-081509.
84. Ilmarinen J. Job design for the aged with regard to decline in their maximal aerobic capacity: part II - the scientific basis for the guide. Int J lnd Ergon. 1992;10:65–77.
85. Fleg JL, Morrell CH, Bos AG, Brant LJ, Talbot LA, Wright JG, Lakatta EG. Accelerated longitudinal decline of aerobic capacity in healthy older adults. Circulation. 2005;112:674–82.
86. Dodds RM, Syddall HE, Cooper R, Benzeval M, Deary IJ, Dennison EM, Der G, Gale CR, Inskip HM, Jagger C, Kirkwood TB, Lawlor DA, Robinson SM, Starr JM, Steptoe A, Tilling K, Kuh D, Cooper C, Sayer AA. Grip strength across the life course: normative data from twelve British studies. PLoS One. 2014;9(12):e113637.
87. Llmarinen J, Louhevaara V, Korhonen O, Nygard C-H, Hakola T, Suvanto S. Changes in maximal cardiorespiratory capacity among aging municipal employees. Scand J Work Environ Health. 1991;17(1):99–109.
88. Nygard C-H, Luopaǰirvi T, Llmarinen J. Musculoskeletal capacity of elderly men and women in different types of work. Scand J Work Environ Health. 1991;17(suppl1):110–7.
89. Nygard C-H, Eskelinen L, Suvanto S, Tuomi K, Llmarinen J. Associations between functional capacity and work ability among elderly men and women. Scand J Work Environ Health. 1991;17(suppl 1):122–7.
90. Syddall HE, D'Angelo S, Ntani G, Stevens M, Harris EC, Linaker CH, Walker-Bone K. Work participation and risk factors for health-related job loss among older workers in the Health and Employment after Fifty (HEAF) study: evidence from a 2-year follow-up period. PLoS One. 2020;15(9):e0239383.
91. Sewdas R, van der Beek AJ, Boot CRL, D'Angelo S, Syddall HE, Palmer KT, Walker-Bone K. Poor health, physical workload and occupational social class as determinants of health-related job loss: results from a prospective cohort study in the UK. BMJ Open. 2019;9(7):e026423.
92. Mackey M, Noone J, Bohle P. Ageing and work ability: implications for promoting healthy working life in an underground coal mine environment. In: Proceedings of the 19th Triennial Congress of the International Ergonomics Association #1886. Melbourne, 9–14 August 2015. http://ergonomics.uq.edu.au/iea/proceedings/Index_files/papers/1886.pdf.
93. van Rijn RM, Robroek SJW, Brouwer S, et al. Influence of poor health on exit from paid employment: a systematic review. Occup Environ Med. 2014;71:295–301.
94. Kang M-Y, Myong J-P, Kim H-R. Job characteristics as risk factors for early retirement due to ill health: the Korean longitudinal study of aging (2006–2014). J Occup Health. 2019;61:63–72.
95. D'Angelo S, Syddall H, Ntani G, Harris EC, Linaker C, Cooper C, Stevens M, Walker-Bone K. How does job dissatisfaction interact with self-rated health in determining the risk of health-related job loss? Prospective findings from the Health and Employment After Fifty (HEAF) study. Occup Environ Med. 2021;78(1):36–42.
96. Ilmarinen J, Rantanen J. Promotion of work ability during ageing. Am J Ind Med. 1999;Suppl 1:21–3. https://doi.org/10.1002/(sici)1097-0274(199909)36:1+<21::aid-ajim8>3.0.co;2-s.
97. Ilmarinen J, Louhevaara V, editors. Finn age-respect for the aging: action programme to promote health, work ability and wellbeing of aging workers, 1990–1996. Helsinki: Finnish Institute of Occupational Health; 1999.
98. Mackey MG, Bohle P, Taylor P, Di Biase T, McLoughlin C, Purnell K. Walking to wellness' in an ageing sedentary university community—a randomised controlled feasibility study WCPT 2011 Amsterdam. Physiotherapy. 2011;97(Suppl 1):eS733.
99. Mackey MG, Bohle P, Taylor P, Di Biase T, McLoughlin C, Purnell K. Walking to wellness in an ageing sedentary university community: design, methods and protocol. Contemp Clin Trials. 2011;32:273–9.

100. Oakman J, Neupane S, Proper KI, Kinsman N, Nygård H. Workplace interventions to improve work ability: a systematic review and meta-analysis of their effectiveness. Scand J Work Environ Health. 2018;44:134–46.
101. Noone JH, Mackey MG, Bohle P. Pilot survey of work ability in Australia: a report to Safe Work Australia: Canberra: Safe Work Australia; 2014.
102. De Preter H, Van Looy D, Mortelmans D. Individual and institutional push and pull factors as predictors of retirement timing in Europe: a multilevel analysis. J Aging Stud. 2013;27(4):299–307.
103. Moore S, Rosenthal D. Routlege women and retirement: challenges of a new life stage; 2018.
104. Wang M. Profiling retirees in the retirement transition and adjustment process: examining the longitudinal change patterns of retirees' psychological well-being. J Appl Psychol. 2007;92:455–74.
105. World Health Organisation. Constitution of the World Health Organisation. Geneva: WHO; 1948.
106. Gorry A, Gorry D, Slavov SN. Does retirement improve health and life satisfaction? Health Econ. 2018;27:2067–86. https://doi.org/10.1002/hec.3821.
107. Fisher GG, Chaffee DS, Sonnega A. Retirement timing: a review and recommendations for future research. Work Aging Retire. 2016;2(2):230–61. https://doi.org/10.1093/workar/waw001.
108. Handley TE, Lewin TJ, Butterworth P, Kelly BJ. Employment and retirement impacts on health and wellbeing among a sample of rural Australians. BMC Public Health. 2021;21(1):888.
109. Baxter S, Blank L, Cantrell A, Goyder E. Is working in later life good for your health? A systematic review of health outcomes resulting from extended working lives. BMC Public Health. 2021;21(1):1356.
110. Sewdas R, de Wind A, Stenholm S, Coenen P, Louwerse I, Boot C, van der Beek A. Association between retirement and mortality: working longer, living longer? A systematic review and meta-analysis. J Epidemiol Community Health. 2020;74(5):473–80.
111. Wu C, Odden MC, Fisher GG, Stawski RS. Association of retirement age with mortality: a population-based longitudinal study among older adults in the USA. J Epidemiol Community Health. 2016;70(9):917–23.
112. Han SH. Health consequences of retirement due to non-health reasons or poor health. Soc Sci Med. 2021;273:113767.
113. Hajdas M, Radomska J, Szpulak A, Silva SC. Don't tell me stories—the narratives of retirement and their relation with brand associations. Int J Manag Econ. 2022;58(1):17–32. https://doi.org/10.2478/ijme-2022-0005.
114. Stephens C, Noone J, Alpass F. Upstream and downstream correlates of older people's engagement in social networks: what are their effects on health over time? Int J Aging Hum Dev. 2014;78(2):149–69. https://doi.org/10.2190/AG.78.2.d.
115. Cherry KE, Walker EJ, Brown JS, Volaufova J, LaMotte LR, Welsh DA, Su LJ, Jazwinski SM, Ellis R, Wood RH, Frisard MI. Social engagement and health in younger, older, and oldest-old adults in the Louisiana Healthy Aging Study. J Appl Gerontol. 2013;32(1):51–75. https://doi.org/10.1177/0733464811409034. Epub 2011 Jun 6.
116. Rowe JW, Kahn RL. Successful aging 2.0: conceptual expansions for the 21st century. J Gerontol B Psychol Sci Soc Sci. 2015;70(4):593–6. https://doi.org/10.1093/geronb/gbv025. Epub 2015 Apr 15.
117. Taylor P, Earl C, McLoughlin C. Australian employer usage of the practice of offering reduced working hours to workers close to retirement: extent and determinants. Australas J Ageing. 2016;35:E13–7. https://doi.org/10.1111/ajag.12253.
118. Douglas H, Georgiou A, Westbrook J. Social participation as an indicator of successful aging: an overview of concepts and their associations with health. Aust Health Rev. 2017;41(4):455–62. https://doi.org/10.1071/AH16038.

Social Connection and Engagement 4

Tessa Morgan and Tessa Pocock

4.1 The Importance of Social Connection and Engagement for Healthy Ageing

Forming and sustaining social connections is widely understood as a deep human impulse reflective of the innate human need to have others with whom we can depend on and trust [1]. This insight has formed the backbone of many academic disciplines including sociology, anthropology, and philosophy [2, 3]. Social connection is increasingly championed as an important public health issue [4]. Furthermore, social connection and engagement are increasingly proposed in policy as ways to promote healthy ageing and enable community-living older people to flourish in their homes and communities for as long as possible [5, 6]. The focus on social connection and engagement aligns with the shift to positive, strengths-based approaches in ageing research. These approaches challenge ageist assumptions that later life necessarily involves diminished social contact and increased levels of social isolation and loneliness [7, 8].

Healthy ageing is understood as "the process of developing and maintaining the functional ability that enables well-being in older age" [9, 10]. For older people, environments and contexts of ageing play a crucial role in promoting healthy ageing [11]. The mechanisms through which social connection and engagement promote healthy ageing are multidimensional and nuanced [12]. On the one hand, social connection and engagement are considered as indicators of healthy ageing in their own right [13–16]. On the other hand, social connection and engagement are viewed as

T. Morgan (✉)
University of Cambridge, Cambridge, UK
e-mail: tlm32@medschl.cam.ac.uk

T. Pocock
School of Nursing, University of Auckland, Auckland, New Zealand
e-mail: t.pocock@auckland.ac.nz

J. Byles (ed.), *What Matters for Healthy Ageing*, Topics in Geriatric Care,
https://doi.org/10.1007/978-981-96-0462-3_4

elements of a more holistic approach to healthy ageing, which can promote functional ability and physical, mental, and cognitive health [17–19]. For the purpose of this chapter, we consider healthy ageing as a dynamic, multidimensional, and holistic process where social connection and engagement are part of the broader picture.

Social connection is an ambiguous concept itself, often standing in for concepts such as collective self-esteem, social engagement, belongingness [20], social integration, social support [21], social capital, participation, and identification [22]. In this chapter, we consider social connection as "an opposite of loneliness, a subjective evaluation of the extent to which one has meaningful, close, and constructive relationships with others (i.e. individuals, groups, and society)" [23]. It involves feeling cared about, caring about others, and feeling a sense of belongingness to a group or community [23]. As a multidimensional concept, social connection comprises three interconnected components, including (1) structural features, such as the size and proximity of social contacts; (2) functional features, including what kinds of social support are provided (or at least perceived to be); and (3) assessment of the quality of connections [4, 24].

While social connection and engagement contribute towards healthy ageing, being healthy and mobile reciprocally impacts social connection and engagement. Evidence indicates that older people with greater social connections and support experience lower rates of depression [25], decreased risks of cognitive decline [26] and mortality [27], and higher physical activity levels [28]. Health and mobility are also predictive of older people's ability to socially connect, as older people with chronic health conditions [29] and cognitive impairment [26] tend to have lower levels of social connection and participation.

With advancing age and changes in capabilities, having a variety of opportunities for formal, informal, and spontaneous social connection becomes more important [6, 30]. There is an increasing focus on broader environmental connection and engagement [6]. For example, policy documents have signalled the role of age-friendly settings and environments in supporting older people's social connection [5, 6]. Furthermore, studies have considered how features of the built and natural environment, such as walkable footpaths [30, 31], availability of public parks and beaches [32], and accessible and affordable public transport [33, 34] facilitate social connection and healthy ageing in general. Increasingly, studies are also considering the ways poverty and inequality impact the ability for older people to feel socially connected, both on an interpersonal level and in terms of belonging to wider society [35–38]. Studies have also highlighted the cost of socialising and hosting as a barrier for participation [39].

Other studies have highlighted how explicit and implicit forms of racism and linguistic exclusion impact older migrants' ability to feel connected to their new home nations [40]. Other innovative lines of enquiry have focused on the positive buffering impacts of social connection for marginalised communities. For example, a longitudinal study with 952 older American participants (68% Hispanic and 17% Black) from low-income neighbourhoods, found that social connections offer a buffering effect for people facing daily adversity and in turn protect against cognitive decline [26]. Another study identified that for older migrants living in Aotearoa,

New Zealand, social participation and connection frequently took the form of volunteering and caring for their community in order to foster a sense of belonging in their new home [41].

Some attention has also been given to the way gender shapes older people's social connectivity [42]. There is some evidence that older people prefer to socialise with those from similar cultural backgrounds [43] and genders [44] where they share taken-for-granted social customs, knowledge, and activities. Studies have highlighted how older women are more likely to be socially engaged in later life, for example, through greater participation in places of religious worship [14]. Nevertheless, older women often score lower on perceived feelings of social connection despite the number of social contacts they have [45]. Studies are also beginning to consider social connection as a broader concept, highlighting that spending time in nature and gardens [32], reminiscing and cultivating positive memories [46], and spending time by oneself [47] are also meaningful alternatives to interpersonal connection.

This section has demonstrated the centrality of social connection to healthy ageing while acknowledging that older people have different social needs and experiences. We have also highlighted many avenues to further understand the impact of social identity on social connection and its relation to healthy ageing.

4.2 The Problem with Loneliness

As stated above, loneliness is frequently conceptualised as the opposite to social connection [23]. The high rate of loneliness among older people has been viewed as a major public health issue [27], long before the COVID-19 pandemic brought the problem of loneliness front and centre [48]. Loneliness is broadly understood as a negative feeling arising from a perceived discrepancy between a person's desired and achieved social relations [49]. Loneliness is often conflated with social isolation, but they ought to be viewed as distinct categories given the former focuses on the qualitative aspects, whereas the latter is concerned with the number of social contacts [50]. Robust evidence links loneliness with increased rates of mental health and cardiovascular issues [27], stroke [51], and mortality [50, 52]. A recent meta-analysis of studies conducted in high income countries, concluded that loneliness affects one in four older people, with higher rates exhibited as people age [53].

Loneliness is considered a problem in older age as this age group are disproportionately exposed to age-related risk factors, such as living alone or in residential care, being widowed, and experiencing chronic illness [54]. These high rates of loneliness are only mirrored in the under 25-year-old population, leading Victor and Bowling [55] to identify the U-shaped distribution of loneliness. More recently, a cross-sectional nationally representative survey from the United States ($N = 2477$) found that the predictors of loneliness, such as household income, household size, marital status, health, and frequency of socialising, did not differ due to age of respondents [56]. The authors contend that this is because age is a broad construct that can be understood as a proxy for a variety of other factors, such as experiences (e.g. major life events), material resources (e.g. income), and non-material resources (e.g. health) [56].

There has been a notable shift to think about loneliness as arising from missing resources and lacking competencies, rather than individual deficits or misaligned social expectations [57, 58]. Resources can exist on an individual level (e.g. income/wealth) or broader environmental level (e.g. accessibility to and views about neighbourhood and community). Non-material resources are also relevant, including communication skills (including digital literacy), social skills (including cognition), and comprehension skills. There is also a shift in loneliness studies to explore the multidimensional nature of reasons for, and experiences of, this complex emotion, particularly through the use of qualitative research drawing on older people's perspectives [59–61]. For example, an in-depth qualitative study with 35 older people living in Tel Aviv highlighted the wide range of reasons for loneliness, which included psychological concerns such as shame and fear of rejection, physical concerns such as mobility, vision and hearing and cognitive decline, as well as external factors such as finances and having the ability to socialise with families living across the world [59]. Overall, there is a strong evidence base emphasising the importance of promoting social connection to buffer against loneliness and work towards healthy ageing.

4.2.1 Successful Strategies to Help Connect Older People

While there is strong evidence around the need to foster social connection to mitigate loneliness, interventions to achieve these aims often remain inconclusive or ineffective [62–64]. This is despite the wide array of interventions trailed so far, including one-on-one, group, and wider community engagement initiatives [62]. Reasons for the limited success of interventions to date largely centre around the lack of integration and adjustment of interventions to fit "the right person, at the right time" [65].

Scholars have identified the following pressing gaps in the literature that perpetuate the misfit of interventions:

- Incorrectly assuming loneliness and social connection are homogenous constructs [65]
- Not targeting individuals' needs and contexts. For example, initiatives tend to propose a single intervention or provide a "one size fits all" approach [66]
- Lack of consideration of wider structural processes when implementing interventions, including consideration of the cultural context [23, 37]
- Overlooking the fact that loneliness and social connection are both complex concepts which affect many domains of life [59]
- Overreliance on quantitative, cross-sectional, correlational studies lacking in any theoretical engagement [62]

Another persistent issue relates to ambiguity around what aspect of social connection these interventions are aiming to address. For example, interventions could aim to increase the number of social contacts people have, increase the range of relationships and social activities people are involved in, or improve the quality of relations [54].

Recognising the issues with the current evidence base, the following sections will critically consider three strategies that organisations and policymakers frequently use to facilitate older people's social connection and engagement. These strategies cover befriending services, digital social technologies, and the contribution of neighbourhood environment and mobility.

4.3 Strategy One: Befriending Services

Befriending is a widely used organisation-led strategy which is employed to increase older people's social networks [67]. Befriending is described as "a relationship between two or more individuals which is initiated, supported and monitored by an agency that has defined one or more parties as likely to benefit" [68]. It is a direct form of formalised and targeted intervention to alleviate loneliness through supported socialisation [66]. Befriending can be conducted one-to-one or in groups, over the phone or in person, at home or through "going out" [67]. Befriending differs from other forms of peer support, such as mentoring, as it develops more informally and organically, and often over a longer period of time [69].

In a recent New Zealand-based study involving 76 ethnically diverse older people and 30 service providers, the authors concluded that one-on-one befriending could be successful when a match went beyond a transactional "professional-client" relationship to resemble genuine friendship, underpinned by mutual interests, reciprocity, and reliability [70]. The importance of mutuality and reciprocity has been identified in other studies [59]. For example, a systematic review of studies with older adult caregivers found peer support to be particularly effective when participants felt they developed a special friendship with someone who would listen to them unconditionally [71]. On the other hand, a United Kingdom-based intervention matching school-aged children with rest home residents over Zoom identified mutuality as a key barrier [72]. The authors noted that younger people often did not know what to say to older people and often required prompting from researchers [72].

Befriending services have also been identified as successful when they connect older people with their culture. Culturally specific group bonding has been identified as important because it is based on shared goals and experiences. The New Zealand-based befriending study mentioned above identified numerous, albeit implicit, suggestions that cultural matching for Māori, Pacific, and Asian participants mattered because of language and cultural understandings of reciprocity and connection [70]. Participants from minoritised backgrounds also tended to express a preference for group, rather than one-on-one, modes of befriending. An intervention study in Hong Kong identified older people's preference for group-based socialising which centred around physical activities aligned with cultural preferences, such as volleyball and Tai Chi [73]. It is important to recognise that group-based befriending takes time and emotional involvement for people to feel connected to a wider group. Furthermore, it is important to not assume that cultural similarities will always result in deep connections [24]. From the established evidence base, variety and choice appear to be important considerations for interventions designed to facilitate friendship among older people. Ultimately more research is required around the accessibility, acceptability, and efficacy of befriending interventions which support culturally diverse communities of older people [74].

4.4 Strategy Two: Digital Social Technologies

Technology has been lauded as a solution to a range of challenges presented by ageing populations [75–77], including improving older people's social connection and engagement [78]. The use of technology can help enhance social connection and increase social support among older people [24, 79, 80]. Technology is characterised as a complement, alternative, and substitute for in-person communication [24]. The benefits of technology for connectivity have been particularly pronounced under COVID-19 lockdown or stay-at-home measures where older people have been home-bound [81, 82]. In addition, particular populations, such as older people living rurally with limited social support services, are also considered disproportionate benefactors of the digital shift [24].

A systematic review identified eight types of technological interventions to improve older people's social connection and/or loneliness [83]. These interventions included: general information and communication technologies (ICTs; email, the internet); video games; robotics; personal reminder information and social management system; asynchronous peer support chat rooms; social network sites; Tele-Care; and 3D virtual environments [83]. Evidence regarding the effect of technologies applied to alleviate loneliness or social isolation are mixed and are currently limited in how they have taken users' specific contextual and individual characteristics into account [83]. Similarly, an evaluation of technology-based interventions found that technology provides a feasible way of enhancing social connections, but can also have an unintended consequence of increasing perceptions of loneliness [80]. Older people's suggestions for improving the success of such interventions involve personalising and matching interventions with users' needs and interests, providing intervention/technology options and allowing users to experiment with these, and ensuring opportunities for meaningful interaction within and across generations [80].

A particularly promising technological area is the use of ICTs to alleviate loneliness and social isolation by facilitating social interaction with family, friends, or volunteers [83]. For example, one study conducted in the United States found that 90% of their older person sample expressed greater connection to their families or the world when using tablet devices [84]. Tablets enabled older people to connect with their families beyond telephone calls, interact face-to-face through video-calling applications of FaceTime or Skype, use digital media or email to coordinate social events with family and friends, and connect with the wider world through e-book, news, weather, or information searching apps [84]. Another study concluded that ICTs positively improved older people's social support, social connection, and social isolation although the impact on loneliness was inconclusive [85]. Another intervention study involving a Zoom quiz across three British care homes found that the intervention alleviated situational loneliness and increased social connections, especially by the interactions involved prior to and after the quiz [86]. While promising, there remains room for future interventions to distinguish between what positive benefits come from technology and what stem from the human interactions around them.

This quandary is most apparent in another technological solution: use of robotic pets to address loneliness. Robotic pets have been found to decrease loneliness in seven intervention studies [83]. This type of technology assists in providing a sense of social presence and communication or acting as a conversation agent [87]. For example, a randomised control trial conducted in Auckland, New Zealand included 40 residents from a residential care facility and hospital in a 12-week programme. This programme involved group sessions with a robotic seal and provided older people with something to talk about, rather than the social connection resulting from the resident and the robot [88]. We contend that these studies might play into the "anything is better than nothing" approach, especially given that much of the robotic companionship studies have been conducted with nursing home residents whose baseline loneliness rates are already low to begin with [83].

It is also important to consider that numerous factors contribute towards the digital exclusion of older people, including socioeconomic and demographic inequalities in technology and internet access, limited digital literacy, language barriers, disability, and lack of desire to access online environments [81, 89, 90]. Concerns have also been raised about the prevalence of the digital divide whereby those living in nursing homes are excluded from access and/or support to use such technology [59]. There is also a concern around whether pushing for technological solutions is culturally appropriate. In a study with 44 diverse older New Zealanders experiencing lockdown, the authors found that technology use was contrary to cultural preferences to communicate face to face [91]. For technology-based interventions to effectively enhance social connection and reduce loneliness, interventions should be tailored to older people's characteristics, needs, interests, and cultural preferences [80, 91]. Furthermore, additional support is required to increase digital engagement and reduce digital exclusion [81].

4.5 Strategy Three: The Neighbourhood Environment, Mobility, and Age-Friendly Settings

Neighbourhood environments are a key part of the discussion when looking at contexts of healthy ageing [11]. The built environment consists of the entirety of human designed and built places and facilities, including community design, function, and transportation infrastructure [92]. For older people who age in their communities, the neighbourhood built environment becomes the platform for social connection, meaningful engagement, and mobility [18]. The relationship between neighbourhood built environment, social connection, engagement, and mobility is complex. First, neighbourhood environments contribute towards health and well-being of older people by providing spaces for social connection and mobility to occur [34, 93, 94]. Second, perceived social connection and built environment supportiveness can influence older people's mobility patterns [95, 96]. And third, mobility itself facilitates social connection and engagement in the environment [30, 96].

The built environment provides sites for formal, informal, and spontaneous social connection and engagement. Considerable literature has focused on neighbourhood third places and transitory zones as key facilitators of older people's social connection and community engagement [93, 96–99]. Third places (e.g. informal, accessible spaces outside home and work such as cafés) and transitory zones (e.g. places passed through in daily life such as seats on buses and public benches) support older people's physical needs by providing an opportunity for rest and support of chronic disease or mobility impairments, while also caring for social needs by presenting a setting for organic development of social connections [97–99]. A further example of neighbourhood sites of social connection and engagement comes in the form of community libraries. In the context of the global COVID-19 pandemic, Lenstra et al. [100] evaluated how small and rural public libraries in the United States continued to support social connections for older people. Among different approaches to supporting social connections, library staff facilitated meaningful opportunities for older people to engage in programmes outside of the library, volunteer in the community, and participate in physically distanced or virtual programmes inside the library. Thus, to increase opportunities for formal, informal, and spontaneous social connection and engagement, proximity to a variety of community resources and social spaces is important [34, 93].

In a recent review on conceptualising healthy ageing, mobility was identified as a fundamental concept which facilitated social connection and engagement in meaningful activities [18]. Physical mobility is defined as movement across space and time through diverse movement mechanisms [101]. For older people living in the community, physical mobility and motility (an individual's capacity to move) are crucial for accessing neighbourhood facilities and play an important part in older people's patterns of social connection and engagement [33, 96, 102]. While mobility facilitates social connection and engagement, personal factors and decisions provide a reason for older people to be mobile in the first place. For example, loneliness can be a significant factor in the decision to leave the home, as can the desire to connect with others [38, 96]. However, mobility choices are affected by numerous factors, including inequitable access and experience over the lifespan [103], loss of a driver's licence [102], public transportation accessibility [33, 34], seasonality [30, 33, 96], and walkable environments [95, 96].

Built environment, transportation, and social connection are considered as part of the strategy to create age-friendly settings. The aim of developing age-friendly settings is to create environments that support healthy ageing and enable older people to maximise opportunities for well-being, independent living, and social participation [5, 6]. Various models of age-friendly settings have been established over the last two decades [104], with the World Health Organization's model of Age-Friendly Cities remaining one of the most well-known [5]. The eight domains underpinning an Age-Friendly City are: social participation; respect and social inclusion; civic participation and employment; communication and information; community support and health services; outdoor spaces and buildings; transportation; and housing [5]. The Age-Friendly City movement emphasises a life course perspective, based on the premise that "age-friendly" design supports the activity of a wide range of other groups, such as young people and people with disability [5, 105]. The shift to considering healthy ageing and social connection in the context of the wider environment demonstrates the multidimensional contributors to social connection. Further research is needed to elucidate the nature of these connections.

4.6 Conclusions and Future Directions

The need for improving avenues for older people's social connection and mitigating feelings of loneliness are well-established. There is increasing conceptual clarity around these concepts though there is a need for such theoretical advances to be translated into intervention studies. This chapter addressed three strategies that organisations and policymakers use to facilitate older people's social connection and engagement: befriending services, digital social technologies, and the contribution of neighbourhood environment and mobility. Overwhelmingly, most interventions to date have focused on enhancing the structural (e.g. increasing network size) and functional (e.g. range of different kinds of social contacts) components of social connections, but were often only successful when they contributed to meaningful, quality connections. Importantly, these connections did not necessarily have to be sustained or prolonged to count as quality and meaningful connections for older people. We conclude this chapter with suggestions for future research directions arranged around the headings of Capturing and Conceptualising and Contextualising and Tailoring.

4.6.1 Capturing and Conceptualising

Further theory-informed research is required to deepen our understandings of social connection and healthy ageing. Avenues for future research include:

- More qualitative research that unpacks this complexity and centres older people in definitions and metrics of social connection
- Clarification around links between healthy ageing and social connection

- Broadening our understanding of social connection by considering the diverse ways older people find meaningful social connection on both an interpersonal and societal level
- Better evaluation metrics for social connection interventions informed by older people's views and experiences of successful outcomes.

4.6.2 Contextualising and Tailoring

There is not a "one size fits all" approach to promoting older people's social connection. Therefore, strategies to enhance social connection should consider structural, functional, and quality components [4, 24] when designing interventions. Furthermore, when designing interventions, researchers, and policymakers should ensure older people have the capacity and power to tailor social connection initiatives in line with their own social needs and contexts. Suggestions for future research considerations are:

- Pay particular attention to socioeconomic and environmental contexts that shape opportunities for social connection
- Critically engage with digital social technologies by considering who has access and how older people want to participate with technology
- Further engage with vulnerable groups of older people, such as carers and older indigenous and migrant groups
- Consider the value of alternative forms of connection, for example, with nature, gardens, and through reminiscence practices
- Ensure we are not simply providing solutions in light of resource restrictions—but rather considering what would result in the best care and connection

References

1. Cacioppo S, Grippo A, London S, Goossens L, Cacioppo J. Loneliness: clinical import and interventions. Perspect Psychol Sci. 2015;10(2):238–49.
2. Putnam R. Bowling Alone: the collapse and revival of American community. New York: Simon and Schuster; 2000.
3. Durkheim E. The division of labor in society (Original 1893) ed. New York: Free Press; 1993.
4. Holt-Lunstad J, Robles T, Sbarra D. Advancing social connection as a public health priority in the United States. Am Psychol. 2017;72(6):517–30.
5. World Health Organization. Global age-friendly cities: a guide. Geneva: World Health Organization; 2007.
6. World Health Organization. World report on ageing and health. Geneva: WHO Press; 2015.
7. Cornwell E, Waite L. Social disconnectedness, perceived isolation, and health among older adults. J Health Soc Behav. 2009;50(1):31–48.
8. Kohli M, Hank K, Künemund H. The social connectedness of older Europeans: patterns, dynamics and contexts. J Eur Soc Policy. 2009;19:327–40.

9. World Health Organisation. Decade of healthy ageing: baseline report. Geneva: World Health Organisation; 2021.
10. Beard J. The World report on ageing and health: a policy framework for healthy ageing. Lancet. 2016;387(10033):2145–54.
11. Keating N. A research framework for the United Nations Decade of Healthy Ageing (2021–2030). Eur J Ageing. 2022;19:775–87.
12. Taylor J. Should old acquaintance be forgot? friendship in the face of dementia. In: Lamb S, editor. Successful aging as a contemporary obsession: global perspectives. New Brunswick: Rutgers University Press; 2017. p. 126–38.
13. Register M, Herman J, Tavakoli A. Development and psychometric testing of the Register—connectedness scale for older adults. D Res Nurs Health. 2011;34(1):60–72.
14. Willie-Tyndale D, Holder-Nevins D, Mitchell-Fearon K, James K, Laws H, Waldron N, et al. Participation in social activities and the association with socio-demographic and health-related factors among community-dwelling older adults in Jamaica. J Cross Cult Gerontol. 2016;31(4):427–47.
15. Wang W, Wu L, Zhang W, Tsay R. Culturally-specific productive engagement and self-rated health among Taiwanese older adults. Soc Sci Med. 2019;229:79–86.
16. Everard K, Lach H, Fisher E, Baum M. Relationship of activity and social support to the functional health of older adults. J Gerontol B. 2000;55(4):S208–S12.
17. Hung L, Kempen G, De Vries N. Cross-cultural comparison between academic and lay views of healthy ageing: a literature review. Ageing Soc. 2010;30(8):1373–91.
18. Pocock T, Woodward A, Wiles J, Raphael D, Smith M. Diverse approaches to conceptualising positive ageing: a scoping review. N Z J Soc Sci Online: Kotuitui. 2022;18(1):1–26.
19. Cosco T, Prina A, Perales J, Stephan B, Brayne C. Lay perspectives of successful ageing: a systematic review and meta-ethnography. BMJ Open. 2013;3(6):1–9.
20. Register M, Scharer K. Connectedness in community-dwelling older adults. West J Nurs Res. 2010;32(4):462–79.
21. Cohen S. Social relationships and health. Am Psychol. 2004;59:676–84.
22. Haslam C, Cruwys T, Haslam A, Jetten J. Social connectedness and health. In: Encyclopedia of geropsychology. Cham: Springer; 2015. p. 1–11.
23. O'Rourke H, Sidani S. Definition, determinants, and outcomes of social connectedness for older adults: a scoping review. J Gerontol Nurs. 2017;43(7):43–52.
24. Suragarn U, Hain D, Pfaff G. Approaches to enhance social connection in older adults: an integrative review of literature. Aging Health Res. 2021;1(3):1–9.
25. Cruwys T, Dingle G, Haslam C, Haslam S, Jetten J, Morton T. Social group memberships protect against future depression, alleviate depression symptoms and prevent depression relapse. Soc Sci Med. 2013;98:179–86.
26. Gardener H, Levin B, DeRosa J, Rundek T, Wright C, Elkind M, et al. Social connectivity is related to mild cognitive impairment and dementia. J Alzheimers Dis. 2022;84(4):1811–20.
27. Leigh-Hunt N, Bagguley D, Bash K, Turner V, Turnball S, Valtorta N, et al. An overview of systematic reviews on the public health consequences of social isolation and loneliness. Public Health. 2017;152:157–71.
28. Smith G, Banting L, Eime R, O'Sullivan G, van Uffelen J. The association between social support and physical activity in older adults: a systematic review. Int J Behav Nutr Phys Act. 2017;14(56):1–21.
29. Adamson J, Lawlor D, Ebrahim S. Chronic diseases, locomotor activity limitation and social participation in older women: cross sectional survey of British women's heart and health study. Age Ageing. 2004;33(3):293–8.
30. Bacsu J, Jeffery B, Abonyi S, Johnson S, Novik N, Martz D, et al. Healthy aging in place: perceptions of rural older adults. Educ Gerontol. 2014;40(5):327–37.
31. Rantakokko M, Iwarsson S, Vahaluoto S, Portegijs E, Viljanen A, Rantanen T. Perceived environmental barriers to outdoor mobility and feelings of loneliness among community-dwelling older people. J Gerontol Biol Sci Med Sci. 2014;69:1562–8.

32. Finlay J, Franke T, McKay H, Sims-Gould J. Therapeutic landscapes and wellbeing in later life: impacts of blue and green spaces for older adults. Health Place. 2015;34:97–106.
33. Peace S. Social interactions in public spaces and places: a conceptual overview. In: Rowles GD, Bernard M, editors. Environmental gerontology: making meaningful places in old age. New York: Springer; 2013. p. 25–49.
34. Levasseur M, Généreux M, Bruneau J-F, Vanasse A, Chabot E, Beaulac C, et al. Importance of proximity to resources, social support, transportation and neighborhood security for mobility and social participation in older adults: results from a scoping study. BMC Public Health. 2015;15:503.
35. Umberson D, Montez J. Social relationships and health: a flashpoint for health policy. J Health Soc Behav. 2010;51:S54–66.
36. Lee J, Hong J, Zhou Y, Robles G. The relationships between loneliness, social support, and resilience among Latinx immigrants in the United States. Clin Soc Work J. 2020;48(1):99–109.
37. Weldrick R, Grenier A. Social isolation in later life: extending the conversation. Can J Aging. 2018;37:76–83.
38. Morgan T, Wiles J, Park H-J, Moeke-Maxwell T, Dewes O, Black S, et al. Social connectedness: what matters to older people. Ageing Soc. 2021;41(5):1126-44.
39. Ibrahim R, Abolfathi-Momtaz Y, Hamid T. Social isolation in older Malaysians: prevalence and risk factors. Psychogeriatrics. 2013;13:71–9.
40. Park H-J, Morgan T, Wiles J, Gott M. Lonely ageing in a foreign land: social isolation and loneliness among older Asian migrants in New Zealand. Health Soc Care Community. 2018;27(3):740–7.
41. Wright-St Clair V, Nayar S, Kim H, Wang S-M, Kaur-Sodhi S, Chung A, et al. Late-life Asian immigrants managing wellness through contributing to socially embedded networks. J Occup Science. 2018;25(1):51–64s.
42. Townsend K, McWhirter B. Connectedness: a review of the literature with implications for counseling, assessment, and research. J Couns Dev. 2005;83:191–201.
43. Nguyen H, Lee J, Sorkin D, Gibbs L. "Living happily despite having an illness": perceptions of healthy aging among Korean American, Vietnamese American, and Latino older adults. Appl Nurs Res. 2019;48:30–6.
44. Franke T, Sims-Gould J, Nettlefold L, Ottoni C, McKay H. "It makes me feel not so alone": features of the Choose to Move physical activity intervention that reduce loneliness in older adults. BMC Public Health. 2021;21(312):1–15.
45. Caetano S, Silva C, Vettore M. Gender differences in the association of perceived social support and social network with self-rated health status among older adults: a population-based study in Brazil. BMC Geriatr. 2013;13(122):1–14.
46. Coleman T, Wiles J. Being with objects of meaning: cherished possessions and opportunities to maintain aging in place. Gerontologist. 2020;60(1):41–19.
47. Dahlberg K. The enigmatic phenomenon of loneliness. Int J Qual Stud Health Wellbeing. 2007;2(4):195–207.
48. Armitage R, Nellums L. COVID-19 and the consequences of isolating the elderly. Lancet Pub Health. 2020;5(5):e256.
49. Perlman D, Peplau L. Toward a social psychology of loneliness. In: Gilmour SDR, editor. Personal relationships in disorder. London: Academic Press; 1981. p. 31–56.
50. Holt-Lunstad J, Smith T, Baker M, Harris T, Stephenson D. Loneliness and social isolation as risk factors for mortality: a meta-analytic review. Persp Psychol Sci. 2015;10:227–37.
51. Valtorta N, Kanaan M, Gilbody S, Ronzi S, Hanratty B. Loneliness and social isolation as risk factors for coronary heart disease and stroke: systematic review and meta-analysis of longitudinal observational studies. Heart. 2016;102(3):1009–16.
52. Christensen A, Juel K, Ekholm O, Thrysoe L, Thorup C, Borregaard B. Significantly increased risk of all-cause mortality among cardiac patients feeling lonely. Heart. 2020;106:140–6.
53. Chawla K, Kunonga T, Stow D, Barker R, Craig D, Hanratty B. Prevalence of loneliness amongst older people in high-income countries: a systematic review and meta-analysis. PLoS One. 2021;16(7):e0255088.

54. Holt-Lunstad J. The potential public health relevance of social isolation and loneliness: prevalence, epidemiology, and risk factors. Public Policy Aging Rep. 2017;27(4):127–30.
55. Victor C, Bowling A. A longitudinal analysis of loneliness among older people in Great Britain. J Psychol. 2012;146:313–31.
56. Hawkley L, Buecker S, Kaiser T, Luhmann M. Loneliness from young adulthood to old age: explaining age differences in loneliness. Int J Behav Dev. 2022;46(1):39–49.
57. Tesch-Roemer C, Huxhold O. Social isolation and loneliness in old age. Oxford: Oxford Research Encyclopedias; 2019. p. 1–25.
58. Dahlberg L. Loneliness during the COVID-19 pandemic. Aging Ment Health. 2021;25(7):1161–4.
59. Cohen-Mansfield J, Eisner R. The meanings of loneliness for older persons. Aging Ment Health. 2020;24(4):564–74.
60. Stanley M, Moyle W, Ballantyne A, Jaworski K, Corlis M, Oxlade D, Stoll A, Young B. 'Nowadays you don't even see your neighbours': loneliness in the everyday lives of older Australians. Health Soc Care Community. 2010;18:407–14.
61. Morgan T, Wiles J, Moeke-Maxwell T, Black S, Park H-J, Dewes O, et al. 'People haven't got that close connection': meanings of loneliness and social isolation to culturally diverse older people. Aging Health. 2019;24(10):1627–35.
62. O'Rourke H, Collins L, Sidani S. Interventions to address social connectedness and loneliness for older adults: a scoping review. BMC Geriatr. 2018;18(214):1–13.
63. Masi C, Chen H-Y, Hawkley L, Cacioppo J. A meta-analysis of interventions to reduce loneliness. Personal Soc Psychol Rev. 2011;15:219–66.
64. Cohen-Mansfield J, Perach R. Interventions for alleviating loneliness among older persons: a critical review. Am J Health Promot. 2015;29:109–25.
65. Akhter-Khan S, Au R. Why loneliness interventions are unsuccessful: a call for precision health. Adv Geriatr Med Res. 2020;2(3):1–24.
66. Mann F, Bone J, Lloyd-Evans B, Frerichs J, Pinfold V, Ma R, et al. A life less lonely: the state of the art in interventions to reduce loneliness in people with mental health problems. Soc Psychiatry Psychiatr Epidemiol. 2017;52(6):627–38.
67. Moriarty J, Manthorpe J. The diversity of befriending by, and of, older people. Work Older People. 2017;21(2):63–71.
68. Joseph Rowntree Foundation. The role and impact of befriending. York: Joseph Rowntree Foundation; 1998.
69. Asada Y, Abel H, Skedgel C, Warner G. On effective graphic communication of health inequality: considerations for health policy researchers. Milbank Q. 2017;95(4):801–35.
70. Wiles J, Morgan T, Moeke-Maxwell T, Black S, Park H-J, Dewes O, et al. Befriending services for culturally diverse older people. J Gerontol Soc Work. 2019;62(7):776–93.
71. Velloze I, Jester D, Jeste D, Mausbach B. Interventions to reduce loneliness in caregivers: an integrative review of the literature. Psychiatry Res. 2022;311(114508):1–10.
72. Zamir S, Hennessy C, Taylor A, Jones R. Feasibility of school students Skyping care home residents to reduce loneliness. Comput Hum Behav Rep. 2021;3:1–34.
73. Leung K, Chung P-K, Chan A, Ransdell L, Siu P, Sun P, et al. Promoting healthy ageing through light volleyball intervention in Hong Kong: study protocol for a randomised controlled trial. BMC Sports Sci Med Rehab. 2020;12(6):1–8.
74. Gardiner C, Geldenhuys G, Gott M. Interventions to reduce social isolation and loneliness among older people: an integrative review. Health Soc Care Community. 2018;26(2):147–57.
75. World Health Organisation. WHO Guidelines on integrated care for older people (ICOPE). Geneva: World Health Organisation; 2017.
76. Biehl J, Moran-Thomas A. Symptom: subjectivities, social ills, technologies. Ann Rev Anthropol. 2009;38:267–88.
77. Xiong X. Bring technology home and stay healthy: the role of fourth industrial revolution and technology in improving the efficacy of health care spending. Technol Forecast Soc Change. 2021;165(120556):1–6.

78. Chopik W. The benefits of social technology use among older adults are mediated by reduced loneliness. Cyberpsychol Behav Soc Netw. 2016;19(9):551–6.
79. Yu RP, McCammon RJ, Ellison NB, Langa KM. The relationships that matter: social network site use and social wellbeing among older adults in the United States of America. Ageing Soc. 2016;36:1826–52.
80. Barbosa Neves B, Waycott J, Maddox A. When technologies are not enough: The challenges of digital interventions to address loneliness in later life. Sociol Res Online. 2023;28(1):150–70.
81. Age UK. Briefing paper: digital inclusion and older people—how have things changed in a Covid-19 world? London: Age UK; 2021.
82. Morrow-Howell N, Galucia N, Swinford E. Recovering from the COVID-19 pandemic: a focus on older adults. J Aging Soc Policy. 2020;32(4–5):526–35.
83. Khosravi P, Rezvani A, Wiewiora A. The impact of technology on older adults' social isolation. Comput Hum Behav. 2016;63:594–603.
84. Tsai HS, Shillair R, Cotten SR, Winstead V, Yost E. Getting grandma online: are tablets the answer for increasing digital inclusion for older adults in the U.S.? Educ Gerontol. 2015;41(10):695–709.
85. Chen Y, Schulz P. The effect of information communication technology interventions on reducing social isolation in the elderly: a systematic review. J Med Internet Res. 2016;18(1):1–36.
86. Zamir S, Hennessy C, Taylor A, Jones R. Intergroup 'Skype' quiz sessions in care homes to reduce loneliness and social isolation in older people. Geriatrics. 2020;5(4):1–16.
87. Beer J, Takayama L, editors. Mobile remote presence systems for older adults: acceptance, benefits, and concerns. In: 6th ACM/IEEE International Conference on Human-Robot Interaction, Lausanne, Switzerland; 2011.
88. Robinson H, Macdonald B, Kerse N, Broadbent E. The psychosocial effects of a companion robot: a randomized controlled trial. J Am Med Direct Ass. 2013;14(9):661–7.
89. Citizens Advice Bureaux New Zealand. Face to face with digital exclusion: a CAB spotlight report into the impacts of digital public services on inclusion and wellbeing; 2020.
90. Hunsaker A, Hargittai E. A review of internet use among older adults. New Media Soc. 2018;20(10):3937–54.
91. Morgan T, Koh A, Fanueli E, Black S, Wiles J, Moeke-Maxwell T, et al. How socially cohesive was New Zealand's first lockdown period from the perspective of culturally diverse older New Zealanders? N Z J Soc Sci Online: Kotuitui.2022;17(4):518–37.
92. Transportation Research Board. Does the built environment influence physical activity? Examining the evidence. Special Report 282. Washington, DC: Transportation Research Board, Institute of Medicine of the National Academies; 2005.
93. Engelen L, Rahmann M, de Jong E. Design for healthy ageing—the relationship between design, well-being, and quality of life: a review. Build Res Inf. 2022;50(1–2):19–35.
94. Sugiyama T, Thompson CW. Older people's health, outdoor activity and supportiveness of neighbourhood environments. Landsc Urban Plan. 2007;83:168–75.
95. Stathi A, Gilbert H, Fox KR, Coulson J, Davis M, Thompson JL. Determinants of neighborhood activity of adults age 70 and over: a mixed-methods study. J Aging Phys Act. 2012;20:148–70.
96. Gardner P. The role of social engagement and identity in community mobility among older adults aging in place. Disabil Rehabil. 2014;36(15):1249–57.
97. Alidoust S, Bosman C, Holden G. Planning for healthy ageing: how the use of third places contributes to the social health of older populations. Ageing Soc. 2019;39:1459–84.
98. Gardner PJ. Natural neighborhood networks—important social networks in the lives of older adults aging in place. J Aging Stud. 2011;25:263–71.
99. Ottoni CA, Sims-Gould J, Winters M, Heijnen M, McKay HA. "Benches become like porches": built and social environment influences on older adults' experiences of mobility and well-being. Soc Sci Med. 2016;169:33–41.

100. Lenstra N, Oguz F, Winberry J, Wilson LS. Supporting social connectedness of older adults during the COVID-19 pandemic: The role of small and rural public libraries. Pub Lib Q. 2021;41(6):596–616. https://doi.org/10.1080/01616846.2021.1970446.
101. Webber SC, Porter MM, Menec VH. Mobility in older adults: a comprehensive framework. Gerontologist. 2010;50(4):443–50.
102. Neville S, Adams J, Napier S, Shannon K, Jackson D. "Engaging in my rural community": perceptions of people aged 85 years and over. Int J Qual Stud Health Well-being. 2018;13(1):1503908.
103. Adorno G, Fields N, Cronley C, Parekh R, Magruder K. Ageing in a low-density urban city: transportation mobility as a social equity issue. Ageing Soc. 2018;38:296–320.
104. Steels S. Key characteristics of age-friendly cities and communities: a review. Cities. 2015;47:45–52.
105. Biggs S, Carr A. Age- and child-friendly cities and the promise of intergenerational space. J Soc Work Pract. 2015;29(1):99–1.

Lifelong Learning and Healthy Ageing: A Global and Singaporean Perspective

5

Susana Concordo Harding, Leng Leng Thang,
and Araviinthansai Subramaniam

5.1 Introduction

Population ageing is one of the most defining demographic transitions in the twenty-first century. The current cohorts of older adults are generally more educated, healthier, and have greater longevity than their preceding generations. This shapes them as not only passive beneficiaries but active contributors to societies and their communities [1]. Thus, opportunities to maintain and enliven older adults' active participation as essential in the promotion of healthy ageing have gained increasing attention and are being addressed within policies and programmes across countries, guided by international charters of global institutions including the recent UN Decade of Healthy Ageing 2021–2030 (hereinafter the Decade plan).

Among the social determinants of healthy ageing, lifelong learning which fosters functional abilities and capacities of older adults and their communities contributes to a holistic perspective of healthy ageing across the life course. The Decade plan describes lifelong learning as enabling "older people to do what they value, retain the ability to make decisions and preserve their purpose, identity, and independence. It requires literacy, skill training and barrier-free participation, including in digital skills" [2]. Hence, learning and personal growth by building knowledge, experience, and skills are critical drivers for the healthy ageing process, necessitating

S. C. Harding (✉)
International Longevity Centre, Singapore, Singapore
e-mail: susanaharding@tsaofoundation.org

L. L. Thang
National University of Singapore, Singapore, Singapore
e-mail: lengthang@nus.edu.g

A. Subramaniam
Geriatric Education & Research Institute, Singapore, Singapore
e-mail: subramaniam.araviinthansai@geri.com.sg

J. Byles (ed.), *What Matters for Healthy Ageing*, Topics in Geriatric Care,
https://doi.org/10.1007/978-981-96-0462-3_5

investments by both governments and individuals in late-life education and learning opportunities.

Such a continuous lifelong process is essential for functioning. Lifelong learning presents multifaceted benefits to older adults' well-being, including enhancing their independence, autonomy and dignity, workforce productivity, eradication of stereotypes and ageism, cultivation of intergenerational trust, and creation of an inclusive society wherein seniors live, work, and play [3]. Hence, it encompasses *being, becoming, and belonging* and embraces both individual *(being-becoming)* and social *(belonging)* aspects to enable meaningful learning (Kidd, 1973 as cited in Russell, 2007 [4]). In essence, it provides older adults to maintain and understand the self [5] which is aptly captured by the words of Jarvis [6]; "as long as I can continue to learn, I remain an unfinished person—the possibility of more growth, more experience and so on remains—or I am still learning to be me!".

In this chapter, we begin by providing an overview of lifelong learning in relation to healthy ageing alongside the key international charters which seek to promote this agenda. The chapter would then proceed to discuss key studies elucidating associated health outcomes of lifelong learning for older adults across the cognitive and psychosocial domains of wellbeing. This is followed by exploring the lifelong learning landscape in Singapore as a case study, by characterising the relevant policies and practices in place, alongside recent developments. Subsequently, a summary of local literature on the benefits and challenges facing lifelong learning for older adults in Singapore will be explored. We contend that older adults are a heterogeneous population of learners, thus there is a need to address inequities they may face in accessing lifelong learning. Hence this chapter concludes with key implications and recommendations from this perspective for future development pertinent to policy and practice.

5.2 Lifelong Learning: International Directions Amidst a Shifting World

Whilst rapid population ageing, especially within the Eastern and Southeast Asian regions, has raised concerns regarding macroeconomic decline, the Decade plan asserts that continuing lifelong learning accompanied by the promotion and adoption of a healthy lifestyle, rise in retirement age and gender equality, could abate the risks and maximise the potential and benefits of population ageing. Thus, investments in lifelong learning which enables skills acquisition and upgrading, as well as in maintaining health and wellness, are increasingly instrumental for older adults to stay functional and relevant amidst the volatile, uncertain, complex, and ambiguous (VUCA) world of economic and technological disruptions. These are aligned with United Nations' (UN) Sustainable Development Goals 3 and 4 concerning the promotion of quality education and health and wellbeing throughout life [7, 8].

Similarly, amidst the varied policy and strategic approaches adopted towards lifelong learning globally, the UNESCO Institute for Lifelong Learning (UIL) [9] stewards and seeks to advance efforts relating to lifelong learning with its member states and intergovernmental organisations. Its most recent report sets out future-focused vision of education which entails a shift towards embracing a culture of lifelong learning by 2050. Recognising the criticality of lifelong learning during old age, the report emphasises the creation of an enabling environment that acknowledges learning as an innate capability that needs to be nurtured including during later years of life [9].

To this end, a pedagogical approach is deemed necessary to promote lifelong learning among older people that recognises their role in society and contributes to the salubrious representation of ageing. Accordingly, the materialisation of the vision of lifelong learning culture is posited to bring several positive effects across various spheres of society and individuals' lives such as the creation of resilient societies with significant positive impacts on productivity, economic growth as well as enhancement of individuals' health and wellbeing, including that of older adults [9].

Studies globally have discovered and documented positive outcomes of lifelong learning in later life on older adults' overall health and wellbeing, across the cognitive, social, emotional, psychological, and physical domains, with even amplified benefits for vulnerable groups [10–13]. These will be explored subsequently.

5.3 Lifelong Learning and Health Outcomes: Towards Healthy Ageing

Lifelong learning matters as it presents implications on older adults' overall wellbeing and quality of life [1, 14]. Participation in lifelong learning activities enhances older adults' self-rated health independent of formal educational attainment achieved during young adulthood. The mediating effect of lifelong learning activity on self-rated health was sustained even after adjusting for sociodemographic characteristics and major health determinants (e.g. physical activity, smoking), reflecting the universal benefits that lifelong learning provides and regardless of one's starting point in life [15]. However, a study conducted in the United Kingdom found that the initial level of education predicted participation in adult learning with individuals from a lower educational background of high school or lower being less likely to engage in formal education (National Institute of Adult Continuing Education, 2002, 2006 as cited in Sloane-Seale & Kops, 2010 [16]).

Generally, lifelong learning is classified into three forms of engagement: formal, non-formal, and informal learning [17]. Formal learning includes organised learning arranged by educational institutions (e.g. universities and colleges) which involves instructors delivering regular courses, lectures, and workshops, which typically culminate with a certification [16, 18, 19]. Non-formal learning refers to any systematic educational activity which occurs outside of a formal educational system, to provide targeted learning opportunities that vary to specific population subgroups [20]. Both formal and non-formal learning are structured and programmatic. In contrast, informal learning entails the accumulation of knowledge, skills, attitudes, and insights from everyday exposure and experiences of living (e.g. surfing websites, watching television programmes, or reading newspapers) [17, 19, 21]. There has been research on how and to what extent these various forms of lifelong learning influence the various domains of wellbeing.

5.3.1 Cognitive Wellbeing

It has been well-established that cognition is dependent upon brain function which can be enhanced through cognitive stimulation, apart from physical stimulation (i.e. exercise) [22, 23]. Continuous learning is one such stimulus posited to have a beneficial impact on cognitive functioning which contributes to healthy ageing as one ages [24]. A most recent multi-country European study, based on the Survey on Health, Ageing and Retirement in Europe (SHARE), sought to investigate the effect of different types of learning activities on cognitive declination measured in terms of verbal fluency and memory scores [25]. This large-scale and representative study which included a longitudinal analysis of 43,687 community-dwelling individuals aged 50 and above, discovered a strong association between cognitively stimulating non-formal (i.e. education and training courses) and informal (e.g. reading books and newspapers alongside playing crossword puzzles, chess) activities and the delay of cognitive decline, despite over a short period of 4 years and regardless of one's age. This finding persisted even after controlling for socio-economic background, health, and social network variables [25]. Further, a recent systematic review and meta-analysis by Noble et al. [26] revealed that engagement in formal education has a significant positive impact on older adults' Mini-Mental State Examination (MMSE) scores, apart from other domains of wellbeing such as physical functioning, life satisfaction, objective health, and quality of life.

Past studies also attest to the cognitive benefits that lifelong learning endows on older adults. The Seattle Longitudinal Study is regarded as one of the most extensive research studies which explored the development and transitions through adulthood with 500 Group Health members in 7-year intervals between 1956 and 1998. Based on the evaluation of participants' age-related changes including cognitive decline, the study discovered that participants' engagement in an intellectually stimulating and complex environment and maintaining high-level perceptual processing speed were critical variables in mitigating cognitive decline. Conversely, increased cognitive decline could result from limited cognitive engagement [27].

Other studies demonstrated the beneficial impacts of everyday informal learning on cognitive abilities. Wilson's et al. [28] longitudinal study between 1994 to 2001 investigated the association between frequent participation in cognitive activities and the risk of developing Alzheimer's Disease (AD) among 801 older Catholic nuns, priests, and brothers without dementia at enrolment. During an average of 4.5 years of follow-up, findings demonstrated that those who engaged in a significant amount of time in any of the seven information processing-centred activities measured (e.g. playing puzzle games, perusing newspapers, visiting museums, listening to radio, viewing television etc.) had 47% lesser likelihood of developing AD than individuals who infrequently challenged their cognition in such ways. Further, the infamous Nun Study which is a longitudinal examination of 678 Catholic sisters aged between 75 and 107 further substantiates that cognitive decline is not inevitable and that lifelong learning is instrumental for the prevention and delay of dementia and AD symptomatology [29–31].

These studies indicate that sustained mentally stimulating activities through lifelong learning facilitate the adaptability and nimbleness of the mind whilst playing a compensatory role for declines in other areas. Thus, exposure to such cognitive stimulation throughout life helps with the maintenance of cognitive abilities and performance in the ageing process through the development of continuously modifiable cognitive reserves [32]. These afford greater protection and resilience in the face of neurological pathology through neural compensation that facilitates the optimisation or maximisation of cognitive performance by the differential and functional recruitment of brain structures and networks [33, 34]. Healthy ageing in later years is hence enabled through prolonged resistance to cognitive impairments thereby facilitating cognitive functioning despite an ageing brain [32].

5.3.2 Psychosocial Wellbeing

There has been a growing emergence of literature expounding on the influence of lifelong learning pursuits by adult learners on their social and psychological wellbeing [12, 35, 36] which empowers older adults to withstand increasingly complex realities of social isolation and loneliness [1]. Participation in lifelong learning institutions has been reported to enrich social lives through the formation of close interactions and relationships with fellow learners, which includes the provision and receipt of supportive behaviours which manifests positive effects on health [37, 38]. Older adults, especially women, are also able to transcend the traditional role of family caretaker and derive enhanced self-esteem and self-image from continuing their education, as they believe in becoming more intellectually competent, whilst discovering new social roles and status in a supportive environment through such elder learning platforms [39]. The social network cultivated as part of the learning process also serves as a protective factor which guards against the deleterious effects of life stressors and fortify one's mental health [22, 39].

Further, based on the Belgian Ageing Studies which examined 67,560 home-dwelling older adults aged 60 and above between 2004 and 2011, on different aspects of daily life (including their educational pursuits in old age), lifelong learning through participation in a course or training was found to have a positive association with social participation of the older adults. The older learners were more likely to be volunteers, members of social associations and had frequent internet usage indicating that supporting lifelong learning could generate additional social benefits [40] which is consistent with Musick and Wilson's [41] argument that "participation breeds participation".

However, based on the theory of cumulative inequalities, older adults' participation in lifelong learning in later life is varied and stratified due to multiple deprivations [42], especially among the oldest age group, older adults from lower socio-economic backgrounds and with poor physical health causing a learning divide in later life. Hence, it is of paramount importance for educational providers, associations, and social services implementing lifelong learning programmes, to recognise that older adults are not a homogeneous group but are widely heterogeneous who differ by age, gender, educational attainment, marital status, income, physical health, and participation in other areas of life, with each affecting older adults' participation rates in lifelong learning pursuits [38, 40].

Using the Korean Longitudinal Study of Aging data, Chae and Kang [43] further substantiate that individual characteristics significantly determine both seniors' (non-formal) lifelong learning participation and life satisfaction. The study discovered that whilst participation in lifelong learning was critical to older learners maintaining satisfactory ageing, economic status functioned as a critical determinant enabling their active participation in lifelong learning. Further, marital status and health presented significant effects on the life satisfaction of the older lifelong learners over and above their economic status. Thus, the authors argue that basic psychological and social conditions for a stable life in old age are requisites for more active participation in lifelong learning activities which consequently led to life satisfaction and wellbeing.

Furthering the exploration of lifelong learning benefits in later life through the non-formal modality, Narushima's [38] qualitative study with retired Canadian older adults discovered that the health-promoting benefits from non-vocational programmes are associated with psychosocial resources and wellbeing gained through learning. The older learners' enduring interests and their effects, informal social support networks in classrooms, and their awareness of their rights to learn were key beneficial learning outcomes functioning as mechanisms for promoting the development of identity capital (i.e. confidence, coping capabilities, life satisfaction, positive mental attitudes), and social capital through social interactions (e.g. friendships, support network) which compensate for physical ailments in later life.

Hence, the wellbeing that seniors gain from their continued learning was characterised as eudaimonic (i.e. of long-term growth, meaning, and health-driven) rather than a short-term hedonic one, which when strengthened by their enduring interests and sustained learning helps the older learners, especially among those with severe health problems, to cope with determination and effort whilst invigorating their positive psychological outlook.

This is congruent with Bandura's [44] promulgation that "Self-management is good medicine", in that "one's self-efficacy to exercise control is a common pathway through which psychosocial influences affect health functioning". However, like Narushima's [38] findings, Hammond [45] notes that only educational experiences which matched adult learners' interests, needs, and strengths provided positive effects on health outcomes through the development of a range of psychosocial qualities including a sense of purpose and hope, competencies, and social integration, apart from self-efficacy.

More recent studies have further investigated the relationship between lifelong learning in later life and psychological wellbeing. Addressing the limitations of her qualitative study, Narushima's [10, 46, 47] subsequent quantitative investigations established that community-based non-formal lifelong learning is significantly associated with positive psychological wellbeing, alongside healthy lifestyles.

In particular, continuous and ongoing engagement in learning displayed through staying in a single course enabled older learners to develop and maintain an informal social support network that helps prolong the resultant psychological wellbeing for the long term. However, the authors acknowledged the limitations arising from the cross-sectional design and methodological challenges due to several probable confounding variables which may have impacted the assessment of lifelong learning on psychological wellbeing, which hinders establishing causation [10]. The authors also did not compare the effects of different types of lifelong learning (e.g. formal, non-formal) on wellbeing.

Addressing such methodological challenges of past quantitative studies (e.g. representativeness, confounding variables), and further comparing and corroborating the benefits of continuous lifelong learning, Jenkins and his colleagues [48–50] discovered through the large-scale national English Longitudinal Study of Ageing (ELSA) which surveyed English individuals aged 50 and above that older adults' participation in non-formal education (e.g. music/arts/evening classes) exerted a significantly larger effect on their subjective well-being than formal education and training courses. The latter was not associated with higher wellbeing.

The authors suggest that compared with formal courses that may have been undertaken principally for work-related purposes, participation in non-formal learning activities like music and in the arts may be more beneficial as they are aligned with older adults' intrinsic interest in and enjoyment of the subject and as they provide an informal setting for socialising and meeting individuals which are deemed essential reasons for learning during later life. Therefore, engagement in such non-formal and leisure-type courses is more relevant and likely to sustain the participation of older adults, thereby improving their wellbeing over time. Indeed, these are consistent with the findings from the literature described earlier. Lastly, the study revealed that although individuals with higher prior education were more likely to engage in lifelong learning (i.e. both formal and informal), without interventions older adults' psychosocial wellbeing is likely to decline regardless of educational background [49].

Exemplifying the multidimensional impact of lifelong learning on older adults' whole-person wellness using the Orientations to Happiness (OTH) framework [51, 52] uncovered those lifelong learners embraced values that promoted multiple dimensions of happiness achieved through the interrelated pathways of meaning, engagement, and pleasure as posited by the OTH framework. The active lifestyle facilitated through lifelong learning fostered older learners' values of maintaining socio-emotional, cognitive, and physical domains of wellness. Further, leading lives of meaning and pleasure were enabled through lifelong learners' value for spirituality which they practised by serving a greater purpose through participation in novel experiences rendered by spiritual or religious organisations. This is especially since spirituality plays an integral role during old age as a conduct of life, whereby help and compassion are intensified, meaning in life is sought for and clarified, contributes to coping with life stressors and subjective wellbeing of older adults [53–55].

The preceding discussion has explored and underscored the central role that different forms of lifelong learning activities have in enhancing older adults' cognitive and psychosocial wellbeing. Whilst it is crucial for countries to embrace a holistic approach towards older adults' lifelong learning across the spectrum of formal, non-formal, and informal learning, the promotion and implementation of lifelong learning efforts are not without challenges and their experiences and extent of successful outcomes differ by country and region based on their respective idiosyncrasies. The proceeding section explores Singapore's approach towards lifelong learning among older adults as a case study from Asia.

5.4 Lifelong Learning from Singapore's Perspective

Despite the burgeoning literature on lifelong learning in Asian countries, most of the extant research has focused on western settings, with relatively limited attention on exploring the interpretations of lifelong learning from the Asian perspective alongside its socio-cultural and political peculiarities [56, 57]. Nevertheless, a noteworthy convergence across countries is the deepening of the neoliberal paradigm adopted for lifelong learning that concerns serving the dominant economic agenda and interests, rather than a democratic pursuit for self-actualisation, especially in Asia [58–61]. Notwithstanding, Singapore provides a case-in-point which has acknowledged and embraced lifelong learning to address both the nation's economic imperatives and the personal learning needs and aspirations of its older adults amidst an ageing population through its policy mechanisms.

Singapore, as a small city-state without natural resources, considers its human resource as indispensable and strategic capital for its socio-economic development [62]. Accordingly, its approach to lifelong learning has been characterised as being pragmatic and as a survival strategy for the country which serves as an economic driver critical for advancing competitiveness on the global front and addressing unemployment locally, thereby urging its people to become lifelong learners [59, 63, 64]. Hence, Singapore had a long history of lifelong learning focused on adult training and workforce development from the early days of nation-building and economic development, which focused on technical and vocational forms of education to upgrade workers' skills and enhance productivity [58]. In this regard, lifelong learning is embraced by policymakers, employers, and educational institutions to aid the workforce, which is increasingly ageing, to stay nimble and flexible in a rapidly evolving knowledge economy [62]. This is buttressed by multiple parallel pathways in Singapore's education system which reinforces the lifelong learning movement [65].

Most recently, Singapore's incumbent Minister for Education echoes this position and the gravity of strengthening workers' continuous skills mastery [66]:

> the success of our education system is not just about churning out 30 to 40 thousand students each year for the job market. It is to do that and support the timely upskilling of 2.5 million Singaporeans each year. Assuming each worker needs to go for significant training every few years, that makes it hundreds of thousands of adults who require upskilling every year. I thought I was setting a high bar, but since then, international experts have told me that we might be underestimating our country's training needs.

Over the years, the emphasis on lifelong learning has been reframed to embrace a wider scope that is applicable to all citizens, young and old regardless of their employment status for the cultivation of an individual growth mindset and a passion for learning [66, 67]. Singapore recognises the criticality of lifelong learning for its rapidly ageing population. Residents aged 65 and above grew from 9% in 2010 to 15.2% in 2020 [68], and this is projected to increase to 25% by 2030 (Ministry of Health (MOH), 2016a). Responding to this demographic shift, the Action Plan for Successful Ageing (Action Plan) was introduced in 2016 as a national blueprint to guide efforts towards enabling older adults to age well in place confidently and gracefully whilst leading active lives within the community. Lifelong learning was identified as one of the key pillars in the Action Plan to promote active ageing among older adults in Singapore [69], consistent with WHO's Decade plan which identifies learning as one of the key functional abilities integral to the healthy ageing process.

Based on a national survey of older Singaporeans aged 60 years and above, engagement in learning was higher among younger seniors aged 60–69 versus those older, with nearly half of them being motivated by job-related reasons [70]. This is further elucidated by the Skills and Learning Study 2017 conducted by the Institute for Adult Learning (IAL) Singapore, which found learning to be positively associated with educational attainment and negatively associated with age [71]. This suggests that the emerging generation of older adults view lifelong learning more favourably and greater efforts are needed to accommodate the growing demand for lifelong learning from the baby boomers' generations onwards [72].

Furthermore, a nationwide study by the National Council of Social Service [73] examined the quality of life of seniors (pre-seniors aged 50–64 and seniors aged 65 and above) by using the WHO's WHOQOL-BREF and WHOQOL-OLD instruments to investigate areas that contributed and needed improvement to their wellbeing. One of the key findings included seniors in general wanting to see improvements in their physical and psychological wellbeing and level of independence. Also, pre-senior workers reported lower quality of life than younger workers across the personal beliefs, level of independence, environment, and psychological wellbeing domains. These were linked to the need for greater developments pertinent to seniors' inclusion in the workforce as well as social participation, including opportunities to acquire new information and skills and engage in leisure and recreation, which will enable them to function well both in the workplace as productive mature workers and participate in the community (e.g. volunteerism). Vitally, providing opportunities for leading a purposeful life alongside recognising their strengths were key to improving seniors' quality of life.

In this regard, motivations for learning by seniors could be categorised as being "instrumental" which relates to work, career and skills training, as well as "expressive" in relation to personal development and social relations [74, 75]. Thus, Mathews and Hwa [76] argue that motivations for lifelong learning opportunities for older adults should be differentiated between older adults still working and looking for re-employment (instrumental lifelong learning) and those who are not (expressive lifelong learning). To this end, Singapore strives to meet the dual needs of having seniors learn and upgrade themselves to stay relevant amidst a shrinking and ageing workforce and technological disruptions, as well as for personal satisfaction and social participation in the community during later life. Employment, social inclusion, and participation in the community are also important contributors to healthy ageing [77, 78], enabled by lifelong learning which serves as a social determinant of health [79].

5.4.1 Key Lifelong Learning Opportunities in Singapore

Lifelong learning among older adults in Singapore is embraced across its formal, non-formal, and informal forms, and driven by coordination and partnerships across every level of society including private and public sectors alongside institutes of higher learning, the grassroots, unions, and civil society. This section will explore various initiatives mooted to engage seniors for lifelong learning, including those spearheaded by the Singapore government as well as community-driven initiatives which help enhance accessibility to seniors.

5.4.1.1 Formal Lifelong Learning Initiatives: Skills-Based and Employability Focused

SkillsFuture Singapore

SkillsFuture was introduced in 2015 as a nationwide initiative accessible to all Singaporeans aimed at both economic development and rendering opportunities to maximise individuals' fullest potential throughout life, regardless of their starting points, through skills mastery. The SkillsFuture Singapore Agency (SSG) under the Ministry of Education, functions closely with government agencies, education and training providers, employers, and unions to ensure that training and upgrading opportunities are readily accessible throughout life [80]. It also serves to enhance capabilities and professionalism of adult educators by guiding the IAL [81].

Since the launch of the SkillsFuture movement, Singapore workforce's training participation rose from 35% in 2015 to approximately 50% in 2021. In 2021, 660,000 Singaporeans were upskilled via the SSG-supported programmes. This is the highest since 2015, partly attributable to the pandemic which provided individuals and employers with the opportunity to upskill [66] alongside support measures like the SGUnited Jobs and Skills package enacted amidst the pandemic for jobseekers [82, 83]. In 2020, 87% of individuals surveyed reported being able to perform better post-SSG-funded training [84]. To this end, the SkillsFuture has been lauded as one of the world's leading lifelong learning policies for its comprehensiveness alongside its strategic and inclusive policy intention [82, 85–87], underpinned by its broad-based approach towards skills development and immense cross-collaboration with multiple agencies as critical success factors [88].

5.4.1.2 Non-formal Learning Courses

The government also acknowledges seniors' different life priorities and potential preference to "learn for learning's sake" [89] through non-instrumental learning pursuits premised upon personal interests, passions, and aspirations [67]. These non-formal learning opportunities are often offered without charge or are heavily subsidised to also accommodate seniors from lower educational or lower income backgrounds.

National Silver Academy

A national initiative dedicated to seniors' lifelong learning exclusively is the National Silver Academy (NSA) launched by the MOH in 2016 and administered by the Council for Third Age (C3A). The NSA aims to offer affordable and subsidised learning opportunities to seniors through its network of post-secondary education institutions and community-based organisations. As of 2021, the network spans nearly 46-course providers rendering more than 1000 courses annually across a wide range of areas that appeal to seniors' interests. These courses are generally more life-skills-oriented, ranging from gerontology, and health and wellness to the arts and IT with 60,000 learning places filled [90]. This also includes exam-free modules which provide seniors with the opportunity to engage in lectures and tutorials alongside regular students who pursue the courses for credit [91].

Digital for Life Movement and Seniors Go Digital Programme

Singapore has accelerated its digitalisation plans nationwide since the launch of the Smart Nation policy in 2014 aimed at infusing technology at the core of the economy, government, and society [92]. This was further hastened by the COVID-19 pandemic, which necessitated that more seniors learn to lead digital lives. To achieve a digitally inclusive society, the Digital for Life movement aims to galvanise the community to "embrace digital as a lifelong pursuit" [93].

The Seniors Go Digital programme by the IMDA was launched to develop seniors' digital capabilities through a three-pronged approach that addresses seniors' skills, affordability, and mindset gap. In particular, digital ambassadors at familiar community hubs such as public libraries and community centres provide one-on-one coaching and small-group learning. The digital literacy programmes are also tiered to suit seniors' learning capacity and help build their capabilities to access basic communication platforms, government digital services and e-payments [94].

5.4.1.3 Community-Driven Lifelong Learning Initiatives

There are several learning programmes organised by community organisations that aim to address the needs and wellbeing of community-dwelling seniors.

The *Young-At-Heart* (YAH!) is the first community college for seniors in Singapore by the non-profit agency known as Montfort Care. YAH! seeks to promote a positive mindset towards ageing and seniors through opportunities for learning and service, whilst developing seniors' self-efficacy. YAH! also encourages older learners to apply their learnings into action by pursuing meaningful work and activities for the community, thereby developing their confidence in their abilities, deepening their personal growth, and expanding their network of friends through the process. For example, the "HAPPY 50!" is a 50-h course, comprising of weekly assignments, required readings and a community project work, through which seniors learn to leverage their strengths and abilities for the betterment of their community and adopt a positive outlook on ageing. The older learners also mark the culmination of their learning journey through a graduation ceremony [95].

Driven by the belief that seniors can imbibe meanings in life through lifelong learning and social networking, *The University of the Third Age* (U3A) Singapore also aims to convene seniors to share life experiences and social-cultural values among themselves including to younger generations. This is achieved through organised activities such as the "SMS Knowledge Café" which encourages peer-led discussions and learning among small groups of seniors regarding topics of interests and concerns of living in an urban community, complemented by educational and nostalgic tours. The "Sandbox programme" empowers senior volunteers to deliver programmatic single or multi-session workshops to a group of senior learners based on topics such as health and wellness, the arts and reminiscence writing. Among the other curated activities include "Seniors-Meet-Youth" programme that aims to connect younger generations with seniors to facilitate exchanges of life stories and values [96].

The *Community for Successful Ageing's (ComSA) Learning Room* developed by Tsao Foundation—a non-profit family foundation aimed at transforming the experience of longevity—provides comprehensive life skills courses and training to assist seniors with attaining mastery in self-care and successful ageing. Participants are foremost guided to map out their own learning journey in specific areas of self-care, which renders a highly personalised learning trajectory to meet their own interests and aspirations for a healthy lifestyle. Courses provided span across various topics of concern such as practising mental fitness, mindfulness, fall prevention, cultivation of positive emotions, and managing and building intergenerational bonds [97].

Lifelong learning could also be leveraged to enable intergenerational bonding by facilitating connections and mutual support between generations, and promoting social connectedness [76]. The Intergenerational Learning Programme (ILP) organised by Fei Yue Community Services' [98] Family Central, matches youth as "young teachers" and seniors in a group learning environment. Seniors could sign up for a variety of practical courses for free (e.g. ranging from digital and social media usage, music, arts and crafts to health management) delivered by students across different schools and institutes of higher learning [99]. Based on a pre- and post-programme evaluation study on the ILP's pilot run, seniors reported enhanced functioning across the mental, social, and physical aspects of wellbeing. Alongside improving seniors' self-perceptions, the ILP programme strengthened intergenerational bonds and positively shifted youth's perceptions about seniors such as overcoming preconceptions that seniors were weak and frail, whilst both generations reported an increase in the perceived age of being old by 5–10 years, post participation [100]. Such lifelong learning modality can be instrumental in addressing ageism by overcoming both external and self-directed stereotypical attitudes.

5.4.1.4 Informal Learning

70–90% of human learning as part of everyday life constitutes informal learning that is self-directed or group determined, which should not be regarded as an inferior form of learning but as forming the basis for an enduring desire and attitude for continuous learning [101]. Everyday experiences such as the use of internet and social media tools as well as watching television serve as a conduit for knowledge acquisition and socialisation [102, 103] although Xie et al. [104] opines that the latter remains a passive technology with limited communication and social interactions with others. In Singapore, 93% of seniors aged 60 and above reported having watched any free-to-air television the past week as opposed to 88% among those aged 50–59 (Nielsen Media Index, 2018 as cited in National Volunteer & Philanthropy Centre (NVPC) [105]). 95% and 58% of seniors aged 50–59 years and 60 years and above, respectively, utilised internet-enabled devices daily [106] amid an increasing trend of older adults adopting technology and participating in online learning [107, 108].

Thus, technological platforms could be embraced for enriching seniors' informal learning experiences. However, recognising that there remains the need to bridge the digital divide for seniors in Singapore, the VintageRadio.sg [109], which is a digital radio service app, was created by former radio presenters exclusively for the silver generation. As part of engaging and educating seniors digitally in user-friendly ways, seniors can informally learn about useful topics such as health and financial literacy or listen to non-fiction materials through multilingual podcasts and audiobooks. Seniors can also relive the joy of yesteryears by listening to veteran long-time presenters leading daily programmes including music that caters to the respective ethnicities in Singapore. More than just a radio station, VintageRadio.sg allows seniors to informally explore digital content in a safe space enabled by easy-to-use features to accommodate those less tech-savvy, which empowers them to start and self-pace their digital journey.

5.5 Impact of Lifelong Learning on Older Adults' Wellbeing: Evidence from Singapore

Despite limited evaluation research, the impacts of older adult learning have been documented in Singapore. Maulod and Lu's [110] qualitative examination of the pedagogical aspects of the courses at the NSA, revealed that the learning experience provided a sense of productivity to seniors and served as a meaningful role substitute which alleviated their social isolation and loneliness and uplifted their self-worth and self-efficacy. The development of such intrinsic psychological resources contributes to the healthy ageing of older adults through positive effects on ageing and health perceptions, which in return influences health behaviours [111].

Similarly, Goh's et al. [70] evaluation of seniors' learning engagements through NSA uncovered personal development or enhancement of "soft skills" as a salient and concrete impact expressed by the study's participants. Apart from being equipped with new skills and knowledge on bettering and coping with physical and mental health, senior learners discovered refreshed perspectives about life in relation to their personal strengths and weaknesses alongside gaining a sense of fulfilment from learning and accomplishing goals. The older learners also associated their benefits from learning with enhancing their social capital through building their social networks during courses, developing skills and knowledge to better connect and strengthen relationships with others including family members and, being able to contribute to the community.

The quantitative component of the study also unveiled a significant increase in psychosocial gains from pre-course to post-course, especially in the areas of motivation to learn, pleasure, self-realisation, civic engagement behaviour, and perceived availability of helpful resources. However, an increase in loneliness post-course was reported reflecting the discrepancy felt from sustained interactions they previously had with course mates [70], which suggests the importance of continuity or augmentation of learning opportunities for older learners. In investigating the influence of seniors' social networks on their engagement in lifelong learning in Singapore, P. Ko [111, 112] argues for the existence of nuances in the social contexts that affects older learners' motivations. Although the roles of kin network (i.e. spouse and adult children) were found to be influential, only children were found to be key supporters whilst husbands' support was construed to be limited. This finding reflected that spousal support intertwines with gender roles in later life, which is essential to and impacts older learners', especially women's participation in lifelong learning. Furthermore, single, or widowed older learners, compared to their married counterparts, drew upon their wider non-kin members and rich network resources to manage their social support, through which they were motivated and shared information on learning courses, reflecting their bridging potential within their social networks.

Further, the benefit of gaining skills through lifelong learning which enhances seniors' capacity also extends to the wider community that seniors participate in. This is corroborated by Singapore's National Volunteer & Philanthropy Centre's [105] nationwide study on senior volunteerism, whereby seniors in general are keen on volunteering opportunities which allow them to cultivate new skills that can be applied to their volunteering pursuits.

Despite Singapore's holistic approach to lifelong learning, challenges exist in its adoption among older adults, alongside areas needing further exploration. According to a nationally representative survey of seniors aged 60 and above in Singapore conducted in 2016/2017, the prevalence rate of lifelong learning was reported as being low with only 1 in 10 having engaged in learning, measured in terms of having participated in at least 1 course or training in the past year [70].

5.6 Looking Ahead: Recommendations for Policy and Practice

5.6.1 Addressing Inequities in Accessibility to Lifelong Learning

The systemic environment of institutions plays an integral role in shaping individual choices and decisions for adult education [113]. Openness of educational systems towards mature students is important to enhance enrolment in adult education. Sweden provides an illuminating case as the Swedish tertiary education is intentionally open to adult learners whilst the labour market legislations support and protect employees who take a leave for study pursuits [114]. The empowerment of mature workers to pursue formal education or learning without job-related concerns, has been found to contribute towards enhanced healthy cognitive function, independence, a sense of belonging as well as increased wellbeing and quality of life [26]. Better educated workers are also found to stay longer in employment and continue undertaking learning courses [115, 116].

Hence, the future of work and its complexity demands a lifelong learning system wherein older workers' adaptability and resilience are strengthened through investments in re-skilling and upskilling opportunities attuned to their unique needs, preferences, and identities, which improves their self-worth dignity and fulfilment. However, such efforts should not exclude other segments of the older population such as older workers in the informal economy, refugees, and migrants as well as those living in remote rural areas [117].

5.6.2 Extending Lifelong Learning Opportunities to Vulnerable Older Adults and Settings

As part of acknowledging the heterogeneity of seniors and addressing inequities in accessibility, older adults from vulnerable groups and settings should be recognised in the lifelong learning agenda. However, the intersection between older adult learning and residential LTC remains underexplored in the literature [118]. Intervention programmes aimed at improving wellbeing of older adults institutionalised at long-term care (LTC) settings often tend to overlook lifelong learning opportunities [119]. Residents of LTC settings, being removed from their local community, often fail to access lifelong learning opportunities made available to those who are ageing-in-place independently [120].

Researchers contrast between third-age and fourth-age learning, in advocating that learning is not dependent on chronological age but characterised as where seniors stand in the extent to which frailty, helplessness, and loss of autonomy is concerned [118].

Studies have exemplified the potential of learning opportunities on enhancing quality of life and wellbeing of LTC older residents as a form of non-pharmaceutical method that improves cognitive outcomes and alleviates agitation, neuropsychiatric and depressive symptoms [121–123]. More specifically, Hafford-Letchfield and

Lavendar [124] conducted a structured evaluation of learning interventions in care settings whereby partnerships were developed between the older persons and community-based learning mentors. Seniors were reported to have experienced profound learning, categorised across different experiences such as acquired learning (e.g. new skills for painting, navigating the internet), application of learning (e.g. investigating health conditions and applying approaches for health promotion), motivational learning (discussing current affairs and sharing perspectives), and learning to support independence (e.g. doing online shopping, maintaining, or creating new social contacts)

Advocating for lifelong learning for persons with dementia (PwDs), Ward et al., [125] evaluated (over 18 months of test period) a pilot study on prolonged educational programmes by a Danish school of teaching and communication, for persons with early-stage dementia. The study found benefits in helping to maintain decision-making, social interactions, and preliminary indications of improvement in cognitive function. Further, Quinn and Blandon [126] advocate for the possibility of learning, new beginning, and becomings even during advanced stages of dementia, defying it as a "wasteland for learning".

Hence, it follows that for lifelong learning to be truly "lifelong", policy exclusion of seniors located in the fourth age needs to be addressed as well [127].

5.6.3 Enhancing Learning Pedagogy for Older Learners

It is vital for learning engagements to be sensitive to older learners' abilities and of those who are differently abled. The following pedagogical approaches have been studied to be useful for older learners: community-based learning in small groups, individual learning or through personalised tutoring from peers, younger generations, or professional instructors [102, 128–130].

A conducive, supportive, and friendly learning environment is also vital wherein the instructors play a critical role. In investigating the strategies used by successful instructors during their engagement with lower-educated older learners within a classroom setting, Ko [130, 131] developed a theoretical model which primarily captured the role of instructors as facilitating a critical process of progressive empowerment of learners. This central process entails three phases which are sequential and incremental yet overlapping and occurring concurrently, the three phases of empathising-engaging to-empowering allows for the gradual declination of the instructor's involvement to facilitate for the final stage of collaborative learning among older learners thereby enabling the progressive empowerment of learners. Maulod and Lu [110] corroborates that the delivery of content in an engaging and flexible manner by instructors entails empowering learners with the choice of toggling between directive and collaborative learning, providing guidance alongside control over some aspects of the learning process, enabling a safe and encouraging environment for exploration and sharing of views, thereby attracting more learners.

Further, theories such as the SOC framework as previously discussed, could be used to guide design of pedagogies suitable for the developmental characteristics of older adults, thereby enabling older learners to learn effectively whilst enhancing their self-efficacy in learning [132].

Finally, amidst the rapid development of digitalisation, the use of technology for learning would increasingly become integral for sustainability of learning. Whilst COVID-19 pandemic encouraged more older adults to get onboarded online, it also deepened the digital divide whereby most seniors experienced varying degrees of challenges in overcoming technological obstacles for digital communication [133]. Thus, greater support structures are needed in the future to enable seniors to be digitally engaged through affordability of equipment, enhancing their confidence, and overcoming their internalised stereotypes about learning ability [134].

Altogether, late-life learning is a necessary continuation of lifelong learning. It broadens the definition of health as including the process of learning and growth which help enrich psychological wellbeing, social inclusion, and empowerment of older learners thereby contributing to the healthy ageing process. Hence, policies and practices across countries need to be targeted and embrace greater sensitivity towards older learners' varied purposes and abilities for learning, alongside accommodating to their health and functional limitations, socio-economic constraints as well as addressing perceived attitudinal barriers from self-directed ageist beliefs which influences their propensity for lifelong learning pursuits. Simultaneously, addressing the environmental structural and institutional barriers is integral to enabling older adults' enrolment and continued engagement in lifelong learning during later life.

References

1. Al Hazzouri A, Elbejjani M, Chahine MA, Sadana R, Sibai AM. Late-life learning and health: challenges, opportunities, and future directions. Lancet Healthy Longev. 2021;2(10):e613–4.
2. World Health Organization. Decade of Healthy Ageing: plan of action. Geneva: World Health Organization; 2020.
3. World Health Organization. World report on ageing and health. Geneva: World Health Organization; 2015.
4. Russell H. Learning for being: an ontological and existential approach. Int J Lifelong Educ. 2007;26(4):363–84.
5. Jarvis P. Learning to be a person—east and west. Comparative education: special issue: dialogue of the East and the West: searching for new perspectives. Comp Educ. 2013;49:4–15.
6. Jarvis P. Learning to be a person in society: learning to be me. In: Illeris K, editor. Contemporary theories of learning: Learning theorists…in their own words. 2nd ed. Abingdon: Routledge; 2018. p. 15–28.
7. United Nations Development Programme. Sustainable Development Goals. The SDGs in action. New York: United Nations Development Program; 2022.
8. United Nations. World population aging 2019: highlights (ST/ESA/SER.A/430). New York: United Nations, Department of Economic and Social Affairs, Population Division; 2019.
9. UNESCO. Institute for Lifelong Learning. Embracing a culture of lifelong learning. a trans-disciplinary expert consultation. Hamburg: UNESCO Institute for Lifelong Learning; 2020.

10. Narushima M, Liu J, Diestelkamp N. Lifelong learning in active ageing discourse: its conserving effect on wellbeing, health and vulnerability. Aging Soc. 2018;38(4):651–75.
11. Narushima M, Liu J, Diestelkamp N. I learn, therefore I am: a phenomenological analysis of meanings of lifelong learning for vulnerable older adults. Gerontologist. 2018;58(4):696–705.
12. Dolan P, Fujiwara D, Metcalfe R. Review and update of research into the wider benefits of adult learning. BIS Res Paper. 2012;90:1–47.
13. Manninen J, Sgier I, Fleige M, Thöne-Geyer B, Kil M, Možina E, Danihelková H, Mallows D, Duncan S, Meriläinen M, Diez J, Sava S, Javrh P, Vrečer N, Mihajlovic D, Kecap E, Zappaterra P, Kornilow A, Ebener R, Operti F. Benefits of lifelong learning in Europe: main results of the BeLL-project. Bonn: German Institute for Adult Education, Leibniz Centre for Lifelong Learning; 2014.
14. Molina MÁ, Schettini R. Lifelong learning and quality of life. In: Rojo-Pérez F, Fernández-Mayoralas G, editors. Handbook of active ageing and quality of life. From concepts to applications. Cham: Springer; 2021. p. 111–9.
15. Yamashita T, Bardo A, Liu D. Lifelong learning, educational attainment, and health outcomes among older adults in the US. Innov Aging. 2018;2(suppl 1):468–9.
16. Sloane-Seale A, Kops B. Older adults' participation in education and successful aging: implications for university continuing education in Canada. Can J Univ Contin Educ. 2010;36(1):1–29.
17. La Belle TJ. Formal, nonformal and informal education: a holistic perspective on lifelong learning. Int Rev Educ. 1982;28(2):159–75.
18. Villar F, Celdrán M. Learning in later life: participation in formal, non-formal and informal activities in a nationally representative Spanish sample. Eur J Ageing. 2013;10(2):135–44.
19. Tam M, Aird R, Boulton-Lewis G, Buys L. Ageing and learning as conceptualized by senior adults in two cultures: Hong Kong and Australia. Curr Aging Sci. 2016;9(3):162–77.
20. de Lima FK, Manuel Pires Teixeira Gil H, Sathler Tavares Batistoni S, Oliveira Costa M, Cachioni M. Lifelong learning activities for older adults: a scoping review. Educ Gerontol. 2022;48(11):497–510.
21. Thang LL, Lim E, Tan SL. Lifelong learning and productive aging among the baby-boomers in Singapore. Soc Sci Med. 2019;229:41–9.
22. Simone PM, Scuilli M. Cognitive benefits of participation in lifelong learning institutes. LLI Rev. 2006;1:44–51.
23. Mattson MP, Magnus T. Ageing and neuronal vulnerability. Nat Rev Neurosci. 2006;7(4):278–94.
24. Abud T, Kounidas G, Martin KR, Werth M, Cooper K, Myint PK. Determinants of healthy ageing: a systematic review of contemporary literature. Aging Clin Exp Res. 2022;34(6):1215–23.
25. Cegolon A, Jenkins A. Older adults, cognitively stimulating activities and change in cognitive function. International Journal of Lifelong Education. 2022;41(4–5):405–419.
26. Noble C, Medin D, Quail Z, Young C, Carter M. How does participation in formal education or learning for older people affect wellbeing and cognition? A systematic literature review and meta-analysis. Gerontol Geriatr Med. 2021;7:2333721420986027.
27. Schaie KW, Willis SL. The seattle longitudinal study of adult cognitive development. ISSBD Bull. 2010;57(1):24–9.
28. Wilson RS, Mendes De Leon CF, Barnes LL, Schneider JA, Bienias JL, Evans DA, Bennett DA. Participation in cognitively stimulating activities and risk of incident Alzheimer disease. JAMA. 2002;287(6):742–8.
29. Snowdon DA. Nun Study. Healthy aging and dementia: findings from the Nun Study. Ann Intern Med. 2003;139(5 Pt 2):450–4.
30. Snowdon D. Aging with grace: what the nun study teaches us about how to lead longer, healthier, and more meaningful lives. New York: Bantam; 2001.
31. Snowdon DA. Aging and Alzheimer's disease: lessons from the Nun Study. Gerontologist. 1997;37(2):150–6.

32. López ME, Aurtenetxe S, Pereda E, Cuesta P, Castellanos NP, Bruña R, Niso G, Maestú F, Bajo R. Cognitive reserve is associated with the functional organization of the brain in healthy aging: a MEG study. Front Aging Neurosci. 2014;6:125.
33. Colangeli S, Boccia M, Verde P, Guariglia P, Bianchini F, Piccardi L. Cognitive reserve in healthy aging and Alzheimer's disease: a meta-analysis of fMRI studies. Am J Alzheimers Dis Other Dement. 2016;31(5):443–9.
34. Stern Y. Cognitive reserve. Neuropsychologia. 2009;47(10):2015–28.
35. Park JH, Lee K, Dabelko-Schoeny H. A comprehensive evaluation of a lifelong learning program: Program 60. Int J Aging Hum Dev. 2016;84(1):88–106.
36. Field J. Lifelong learning. In: Rubenson K, editor. Adult learning and education. Oxford: Elsevier; 2011. p. 20–8.
37. Mehrotra CM. In defense of offering educational programs for older adults. Educ Gerontol. 2003;29(8):645–55.
38. Narushima M. More than nickels and dimes: the health benefits of a community-based lifelong learning programme for older adults. Int J Lifelong Educ. 2008;27(6):673–92.
39. Lamb R, Brady M. Participation in lifelong learning institutes: what turns members on? Educ Gerontol. 2005;31:207–24.
40. De Donder L, Brosens D, De Witte N, Buffel T, Dury S, Smetcoren AS, Verté D. Lifelong learning in old age: results from the Belgian ageing studies. Procedia-Soc Behav Sci. 2014;116:513–7.
41. Musick MA, Wilson J. Volunteers: a social profile. Bloomington: Indiana University Press; 2008.
42. Ferraro KF, Shippee PT, Schafer MH. Cumulative inequality theory for research on aging and the life course. In: Bengtson VL, Gans D, Putney NM, Silverstein M, editors. Handbook of theories of aging. 2nd ed. New York: Springer; 2009. p. 413–33.
43. Chae SE, Kang G. Determinants of older Korean adults' participation in life-long learning programmes and life satisfaction. Int J Lifelong Educ. 2018;37(6):689–700.
44. Bandura A. Health promotion by social cognitive means. Health Educ Behav. 2004;31(2):143–64.
45. Hammond C. Impacts of lifelong learning upon emotional resilience, psychological and mental health: fieldwork evidence. Oxford Rev Educ. 2004;30(4):551–68.
46. Narushima M, Liu J, Diestelkamp N. The association between lifelong learning and psychological well-being among older adults: implications for interdisciplinary health promotion in an aging society. Act Adapt Aging. 2013;37(3):239–50.
47. Narushima M, Liu J, Diestelkamp N. Motivations and perceived benefits of older learners in a public continuing education program: influence of gender, income, and health. Educ Gerontol. 2013;39(8):569–84.
48. Jenkins A. Participation in learning and wellbeing among older adults. Int J Lifelong Educ. 2011;30(3), 403–420.
49. Jenkins A, Mostafa T. Learning and Wellbeing Trajectories Among Older Adults in England. Working paper. DoQSS Working Paper series, DoQSS . Institute of Education, University of London; 2013. https://discovery.ucl.ac.uk/id/eprint/10018762/1/DoQSS_jenkins_mostafa.pdf.
50. Jenkins A, Mostafa T. The effects of learning on wellbeing for older adults in England. Ageing Soc. 2015;35(10), 2053–2070. https://doi.org/10.1017/S0144686X14000762.
51. Peterson C, Park N, Seligman ME. Orientations to happiness and life satisfaction: the full life versus the empty life. J Happiness Stud. 2005;6(1):25–41.
52. Obhi HK, Hardy A, Margrett JA. Values of lifelong learners and their pursuits of happiness and whole-person wellness. Aging Ment Health. 2021;25(4):672–8.
53. Can Oz Y, Duran S, Dogan K. The meaning and role of spirituality for older adults: a qualitative study. J Relig Health. 2022;61(2):1490–504.
54. Janhsen A, Golla H, Mantell P, Woopen C. Transforming spirituality through aging: coping and distress in the search for meaning in very old age. J Relig Spiritual Aging. 2021;33(1):38–53.

55. Piedmont RL, Ciarrochi JW, Dy-Liacco GS, Williams JEG. The empirical and conceptual value of the spiritual transcendence and religious involvement scales for personality research. Psychol Relig Spiritual. 2009;1(3):162–79.
56. Tan C. Lifelong learning through the SkillsFuture movement in Singapore: challenges and prospects. Int J Lifelong Educ. 2017;36(3):278–91.
57. Tam M. Towards a cross-cultural understanding of ageing and learning by senior adults in Hong Kong and Australia. Int J Lifelong Educ. 2017;36(5):565–77.
58. Lee M, Morris P. Lifelong learning, income inequality and social mobility in Singapore. Int J Lifelong Educ. 2016;35(3):286–312.
59. Ng PT. An examination of lifelong learning policy rhetoric and practice in Singapore. Int J Lifelong Educ. 2013;32(3):318–34.
60. Lee WO. Lifelong learning in Asia: eclectic concepts, rhetorical ideals, and missing values; implications for values education. In: Aspin DN, Chapman JD, editors. Values education and lifelong learning: principles, policies, programmes. Dordrecht: Springer; 2007. p. 362–79.
61. Olssen M. Understanding the mechanisms of neoliberal control: lifelong learning, flexibility and knowledge capitalism. Int J Lifelong Educ. 2006;25(3):213–30.
62. Mehta KK. Unlocking the potentials of an older workforce: the Singapore case. Indian J Gerontol. 2020;34(2):243–54.
63. Kumar P. Singapore: trends and directions in lifelong learning. In: Milana M, Webb S, Holford J, Waller R, Jarvis P, editors. The Palgrave international handbook on adult and lifelong education and learning. London: Palgrave Macmillan; 2017. p. 609–72.
64. Kumar P. Lifelong learning in Singapore: where are we now? Int J Lifelong Educ. 2004;23(6):559–68. https://doi.org/10.1080/0260370420003111479.
65. Ministry of Education. Multiple pathways, new opportunities [Internet]. Singapore: Ministry of Education; 2021. Available from: https://www.moe.gov.sg/microsites/cos2021/multiple-pathways.html.
66. Chan CS. Opening address by Mr Chan Chun Sing, Minister for Education, at the SkillsFuture Festival 2022, Lifelong Learning Institute [Internet]. Singapore: Ministry of Education; 2022. Available from: https://www.moe.gov.sg/news/speeches/20220705-opening-address-by-mr-chan-chun-sing-minister-for-education-at-the-skillsfuture-festival-2022-lifelong-learning-institute.
67. Sung J, Freebody S. Lifelong learning in Singapore: where are we? Asia Pacific J Educ. 2017;37(4):615–28.
68. Ministry of Social and Family Development. Ageing families in Singapore, 2010–2020. Singapore: Ministry of Social and Family Development; 2022.
69. Ministry of Health. I feel young in my Singapore! Action plan for successful ageing. Singapore: MOH; 2016.
70. Goh V, Maulod A, Malhotra R. The pursuit of learning among older Singaporeans. Singapore: Centre for Ageing Research & Education, DUKE-NUS Medical School; 2021.
71. Lee WO. Monitoring mechanisms for lifelong learning in Singapore: why, how, and what's more? Singapore: Institute for Adult Learning Singapore; 2019.
72. Thang LL, Leng CF, Yow A, Cai YH. Lifelong learning among older adults in Singapore. Singapore: Fei Yue Community Services; 2012.
73. National Council of Social Service. Understanding the quality of life of seniors. Singapore: NCSS; 2018.
74. Tam M. Later life learning experiences: listening to the voices of Chinese elders in Hong Kong. Int J Lifelong Educ. 2016;35(5):569–85.
75. Tam M. Elder learning in Hong Kong: policies, programmes, provisions, and issues. Educ Gerontol. 2012;38(2):107–13.
76. Mathews M, Hwa TLY. Towards ageing well: aspirations, challenges and initiatives. IPS Exch. 2014;2(September 2014):1–144.
77. Sadana R, Blas E, Budhwani S, Koller T, Paraje G. Healthy ageing: raising awareness of inequalities, determinants, and what could be done to improve health equity. Gerontologist. 2016;56(Suppl 2):S178–93.

78. Oxley H. Policies for healthy ageing: an overview. OECD Health Working Papers, 42. Paris: OECD Publishing; 2009.
79. World Health Organization. Social determinants of health [Internet]. Geneva: World Health Organisation; n.d.. Available from: https://www.who.int/health-topics/social-determinants-of-health#tab=tab_1.
80. SkillsFuture. About SkillsFuture [Internet]. Singapore: Government of Singapore; 2022. Available from: https://www.skillsfuture.gov.sg/AboutSkillsFuture.
81. SkillsFuture. Training and adult education [Internet]. Singapore: Government of Singapore; 2021. Available from: https://www.ssg.gov.sg/wsq/Industry-and-Occupational-Skills/Training-and-Adult-Education-WSQ.html.
82. Sung J, Sheng YZ, Liau AK, Xinhui AC, Liu L, Coates H. Augmenting the role of higher education institutions in lifelong learning: designing an indicator framework for policy application. Int J Chin Educ. 2022;11(1):1–12.
83. Singapore W. SGUnited mid-career pathways programme for mid-career individuals. Singapore: WSG; 2022.
84. SkillsFuture. Building strategic skills for the new economy. Annual report 2020/2021. Singapore: Government of Singapore; 2022.
85. Myers J. This is how Singapore is preparing for the future of work [Internet]. Geneva: World Economic Forum; 2021. Available from: https://www.weforum.org/agenda/2021/09/singapore-future-work-sdis21/.
86. Ra S, Shrestha U, Khatiwada S, Yoon SW, Kwon K. The rise of technology and impact on skills. Int J Train Res. 2019;17:26–40.
87. Oosi O, Koramo M, Korhonen N, Järvelin A, Luukkonen T, Tirronen J, Jauhola L. A study on structures to support continuous learning-international benchlearning. Finland: Ministry of Education and Culture; 2019.
88. Fung M. Developing a robust system for upskilling and reskilling the workforce: lessons from the SkillsFuture movement in Singapore. In: Panth B, Maclean R, editors. Anticipating and preparing for emerging skills and jobs. Cham: Springer; 2020. p. 321–7.
89. Ministry of Health. "Learn for fun, learn for life"at the National Silver Academy [Internet]. Singapore: Ministry of Health and Ministry of Education; 2016. Available from: https://www.moh.gov.sg/news-highlights/details/learn-for-fun-learn-for-life-at-the-national-silver-academy.
90. Mahzam R. Speech by Ms Rahayu Mahzam, parliamentary secretary, Ministry of Health, at the launch of Geragory Guidelines [internet]. Singapore: Ministry of Health; 2021. https://www.moh.gov.sg/news-highlights/details/speech-by-ms-rahayu-mahzam-parliamentary-secretary-ministry-of-health-at-the-launch-of-geragogy-guidelines.
91. Council for Third Age. Exam-free modules [Internet]. Singapore: C3A; 2022. Available from: https://www.c3a.org.sg/exam-free-modules.
92. Ng CK. Digital government, smart nation: pursuing singapore's tech imperative. Singapore: Civil Service College; 2019.
93. Infocomm Media Development Authority. Digital for life. Singapore: IMDA; 2022. Available from: https://www.imda.gov.sg/for-community/digital-readiness/Digital-For-Life.
94. Infocomm Media Development Authority. Seniors Go Digital program [Internet]. Singapore: IMDA; n.d.. Available from: https://www.imda.gov.sg/-/media/Imda/Files/News-and-Events/Media-Room/Media-Releases/08/Annex-A-Seniors-Go-Digital-Programme-Factsheet.pdf?la=en.
95. Montfort Care. Our story [Internet]. Singapore: Montfort Care; 2021. Available from: https://www.yah.org.sg/.
96. University of the Third Age Singapore. Home [Internet]. Singapore: University of Singapore; 2022. Available from: https://www.u3rdagesingapore.org/.
97. Tsao Foundation. Learning room [Internet]. Singapore: Tsao Foundation; 2022. Available from: https://tsaofoundation.org/towards-successful-ageing/comsa/learning-room.
98. Fei Yue Community Services. Intergenerational Learning Programme [Internet]. Singapore: Fei Yue Community Services; 2019. Available from: https://www.family-central.sg/intergenerational-learning-programme/.

99. Council for Third Age. Intergenerational learning programme [Internet]. Singapore: C3A; 2022. Available from: https://www.c3a.org.sg/intergenerational-learning-programme.
100. Council for Third Age. An intergenerational learning program in Singapore. J Intergenerational Relationsh 2012;10(1):86–92.
101. Latchem CR. Informal learning and non-formal education for development. J Learn Dev. 2014;1(1):1–13.
102. Morrison D, McCutheon J. Empowering older adults' informal, self-directed learning: harnessing the potential of online personal learning networks. Res Pract Technol Enhanc Learn. 2019;14(1):1–16.
103. Smith MC, Smith TJ. Low-education adults' participation in informal learning activities: relationships with selected demographic characteristics. Adult Basic Educ Lit J. 2008;2(2):67–73.
104. Xie B, Charness N, Fingerman K, Kaye J, Kim MT, Khurshid A. When going digital becomes a necessity: ensuring older adults' needs for information, services, and social inclusion during COVID-19. J Ageing Soc Policy. 2020;32(4–5):460–70.
105. National Volunteer & Philanthropy Centre. Empowering seniors through volunteerism individual giving study 2018—Silver V Study. Singapore: NVPC; 2019.
106. Tan YX. The Silver Generation in the age of digital disruptions. Singapore: Centre for Liveable Cities; 2020.
107. Fong BY, Yee HH, Ng TK, Law VT. The use of technology for online learning among older adults in Hong Kong. Int Rev Educ. 2022;68:389–407.
108. Infocomm Media Development Authority. Tech adoption on the rise among Singapore residents [Internet]. Singapore: IMDA; 2015. Available from: https://www.imda.gov.sg/news-and-events/Media-Room/archived/ida/Media-Releases/2015/tech-adoption-on-the-rise-among-singapore-residents.
109. Akinola S. Keeping seniors connected through music [Internet]. Singapore: Agency for Integrated Care; 2020. Available from: https://www.aic-blog.com/index.php/Vintage-Radio-SG#:~:text=More%20than%20just%20a%20radio,space%20to%20relax%20and%20enjoy.
110. Maulod A, Lu SY. "I'm slowly ageing but I still have my value": challenging ageism and empowering older persons through lifelong learning in Singapore. Educ Gerontol. 2020;46(10):628–41.
111. Remm S, Halcomb E, Hatcher D, Frost SA, Peters K. Understanding relationships between general self-efficacy and the healthy ageing of older people: an integrative review. J Clin Nurs. 2021; [epub ahead of print].
112. Ko P. Investigating social networks of older Singaporean learners: a mixed methods approach. Educ Gerontol. 2020;46(4):207–22.
113. Kosyakova Y, Bills DB. Formal adult education and socioeconomic inequality: Second chances or Matthew Effects?. Sociology Compass. 2021;15(9):1–15.
114. Hällsten M. Is it ever too late to study? The economic returns on late tertiary degrees in Sweden. Econ Educ Rev. 2012;31(1):179–94.
115. von Werder M, Thum AE. Extending working life in Finland. CEPS Working Document No. 387. Brussels: CEPS; 2013.
116. Golinowska S, Sowa A, Deeg D, Socci M, Principi A, Rodrigues R, Ilinca S, Galenkamp H. Participation in formal learning activities of older Europeans in poor and good health. Eur J Ageing. 2016;13(2):115–27.
117. Akinola S. How can we best engage older workers in reskilling efforts? [Internet]. Hamburg: World Economic Forum; 2021. Available from: https://www.weforum.org/agenda/2021/05/how-can-we-engage-older-workers-in-reskilling-efforts-jobs-reset-summit-ageing-workforce-longevity-upskilling/.
118. Formosa M. Learning opportunities for older persons in residential long-term care: a systematic review. In: Mikulec B, Kump S, Košmerl T, editors. Reflections on adult education and learning: the adult education legacy of Sabina Jelenc Krašovec. Ljubljana: Ljubljana University Press; 2021. p. 109–22.

119. Buedo Guirado C, Rubio Rubio L, Dumitrache Dumitrache CG, Romero Coronado J. Active aging program in nursing homes: effects on psychological well-being and life satisfaction. Psychosoc Interv. 2020;29(1):49–57.
120. Kydd A, Fulford H. Access to learning opportunities for residents in care homes: reviewing the challenges and possibilities. Maturitas. 2020;140:14–23. https://doi.org/10.1016/j.maturitas.2020.05.019.
121. Namazi KH, McClintic M. Computer use among elderly persons in long-term care facilities. Educ Gerontol. 2003;29(6):535–50.
122. Shapira N, Barak A, Gal I. Promoting older adults' well-being through Internet training and use. Aging Ment Health. 2007;11(5):477–84.
123. Buettner L, Fitzsimmons S. Activity calendars for older adults with dementia: what you see is not what you get. Am J Alzheimers Dis Other Dement. 2003;18(4):215–26.
124. Hafford-Letchfield T, Lavender P. Quality improvement through the paradigm of learning. Qual Ageing Older Adults. 2015;16(4):195–207.
125. Ward A, Alberg Sorensen K, Kousgaard H, Schack Thoft D, Parkes J. Going back to school—an opportunity for lifelong learning for people with dementia in Denmark (Innovative practice). Dementia. 2020;19(7):2461–8.
126. Quinn J, Blandon C. The potential for lifelong learning in dementia: a post-humanist exploration. Int J Lifelong Educ. 2017;36(5):578–94.
127. Formosa M. Lifelong learning in later life. In: Schmidt-Hertha B, Krašovec SJ, Formosa M, editors. Learning across generations in Europe. Contemporary issues in older adult education. Rotterdam: SensePublishers; 2014. p. 11–21.
128. Castilla D, Botella C, Miralles I, Bretón-López J, Dragomir-Davis AM, Zaragoza I, Garcia-Palacios A. Teaching digital literacy skills to the elderly using a social network with linear navigation: a case study in a rural area. Int J Human-Comput Stud. 2018;118:24–37.
129. Lawton PH, La Porte AM. Beyond traditional art education: transformative lifelong learning in community-based settings with older adults. Stud Art Educ. 2013;54(4):310–20.
130. Osborne M, Borkowska K. A European lens upon adult and lifelong learning in Asia. Asia Pacific Educ Rev. 2017;18(2):269–80.
131. Ko H. Teaching older adults: an instructional model from Singapore. Educ Gerontol. 2020;46(12):731–45.
132. Leng CF, Lim WL. Lifelong learning among older adults in Singapore: an overview. In: Findsen B, Wei H-C, Li A-T, editors. Taiwan's senior learning movement. Lifelong learning book series. Cham: Springer; 2022. p. 56–66.
133. Seifert A, Cotten SR, Xie B. A double burden of exclusion? Digital and social exclusion of older adults in times of COVID-19. J Gerontol B Psychol Sci Soc Sci. 2021;76(3):e99–e103.
134. Withnall A. A global perspective on later life learning. In: Findsen B, Wei HC, Li AT, editors. Taiwan's senior learning movement. Perspectives from outside in and from inside out. Cham: Springer; 2022. p. 23–36.

Driving, Mobility, and Healthy Ageing

6

Kaarin J. Anstey, Mitiku Hambisa,
and Ranmalee Eramudugolla

6.1 Introduction

Driving is a critical component of mobility and has become a prerequisite for independent living in many modern societies. As global populations experience increased longevity along with improved health in late life, this has also meant that more older adults continue to drive for longer now than in the past. Drivers now aged in their 70s expect to continue driving for a further 12 to 13 years on average [1, 2]. This is consistent with cohort effects observed in many jurisdictions [3, 4]. In Australia, trends in licensing rates for adults aged in their 70s have risen steadily from 75% in 2011 to 85% in 2019, and for those aged 80 and above from 45% to 55% in the same period [5]. Greater access to private transport among older adults brings with it greater independence and is associated with lower rates of disability, reduced social isolation, morbidity, and mortality. However, due to a combination of age-related declines in function and increased frailty, vehicle crash rates, injury, and fatality rates are also elevated in older age relative to middle age [6, 7]. Although chronological age remains a strong correlate of declining driving safety [6], and driving cessation [8], a wide range of contextual and personal factors contribute to an individual's decision to continue driving into late life.

K. J. Anstey (✉) · R. Eramudugolla
The University of New South Wales, Sydney, NSW, Australia
e-mail: k.anstey@unsw.edu.au; r.eramudugolla@unsw.edu.au

M. Hambisa
The University of Newcastle, Newcastle, NSW, Australia
e-mail: mitikkuuf@gmail.com

J. Byles (ed.), *What Matters for Healthy Ageing*, Topics in Geriatric Care,
https://doi.org/10.1007/978-981-96-0462-3_6

6.2 Driving and Social Engagement

Social engagement is important for health and wellbeing and quality of life at all ages [9, 10]. Lack of social engagement, isolation, and loneliness are now understood to impact not only mood and subjective wellbeing but physiological stress, cardiovascular health, and immune function [9, 11] and is a significant risk factor for cognitive decline, morbidity, and mortality [11, 12]. Older adults are at greater risk of experiencing social isolation as they withdraw from regular employment and caregiving, live longer, and with more chronic health conditions [8]. Social engagement in late life can include participation in a range of out of home activities, either productive or recreational—such as formal or informal volunteering, caring for family, participation in religious or cultural groups, sporting or social clubs, hobby groups, peer or family groups, or visiting public places [13–15]. In many societies, urban and suburban environments have been designed with private transport in mind, with facilities and communities spread across distances that require driving but with limited coverage or accessibility of public transport networks [3, 16]. As a result, driving is a key enabler for social engagement [17].

Activities such as volunteering and time spent with others are important predictors of older adults' sense of wellbeing and of life being worthwhile, and this is found both cross-sectionally and longitudinally [18–20]. Evidence also suggests that socially active older adults are more likely to have better cognitive health, mental and physical health, lower mortality, and greater physical functioning. Data from North America, Japan, and Australia indicate the spatial range of everyday activity, or life-space, is typically larger for older adults who drive than for those who no longer drive [4, 21, 22]. Although not synonymous with social participation, higher scores on measures of life-space are associated with better wellbeing [23], mortality [24], health, and reduced risk of social isolation [25]. It is thus an important motivation to maintain driving skills.

6.3 Driving Cessation

A range of factors predict driving reduction and cessation in older adults, including sensory and cognitive decline, physical functioning as well as gender, financial status, living situation, and access to facilities. Most older adults gradually regulate their driving exposure by limiting their trips to local areas, avoiding complex intersections, driving only during daylight hours and in off peak traffic [26]. This self-regulation may eventually lead to driving cessation. Age remains a strong predictor of driving self-regulation and cessation, however, there is evidence this age effect is weakening with more recent cohorts of older adults being 20% to 30% less likely to reduce driving in late life relative to prior generations [3]. In addition to advancing age, factors that predict self-regulation include poorer visual acuity, eye disease, comorbid health conditions, declining cognition, and higher rates of medication [27–30]. Drivers with eye disease have higher crash rates and report greater driving difficulties and are more likely to self-regulate compared to drivers without vision impairment [31]. Cataracts are one of the most common eye diseases in late life, and nearly half of all affected drivers will limit their driving while awaiting eye surgery [32], with evidence that depressive symptoms increase even during this pre-surgery waiting period [33]. Qualitative research has shown that older drivers often attribute their own driving cessation to visual difficulties [34].

Physical frailty is associated with increased age and risk of driving regulation and cessation [30]. Prospective studies indicate that frailty and driving status are independent predictors of disability in older adults such that driving cessation can increase levels of disability in those who are already frail [35]. Cognitive impairment is also consistently associated with unsafe driving and self-regulation. Drivers with mild cognitive impairment (MCI) are more likely to regulate driving than cognitively intact drivers, particularly by avoiding complex manoeuvres such as turning across traffic [36]. While this may reduce risk if these drivers were to progress to dementia, it is worth noting that there is a high rate of reversion from MCI to cognitively normal, and that crash rates and on-road skills are not consistently impaired in MCI relative to healthy drivers [37, 38].

6.4 Older Adults' Self-Assessment and Insight into Driving

The capacity to self-regulate or voluntarily cease driving relies on adequate insight, capacity for self-monitoring, and awareness of the impact of one's health conditions on driving. There is evidence that drivers' self-perception of their own driving quality, and self-rated difficulties do not match with their on-road performance [39]. Similarly, drivers' self-perception of specific skills such as hazard perception do not correlate well with objective measures [40] indicating that older drivers are unlikely to be aware of deterioration in hazard perception on-road. Instead, self-regulation may be driven by a more general perception of health status and feedback from others. Lower self-rated health significantly predicts driver self-regulation and cessation, independently of disease burden [29]. Similarly, high health literacy and knowledge of conditions that impact driving safety are also predictive of self-regulation [27].

6.5 Impacts of Driving Cessation

The impact of driving cessation on older adults and the capacity to adapt to this mobility change is moderated by a range of sociodemographic factors. These factors can further compound health disparities in late life. Gender has a significant influence on decisions to reduce or stop driving in late life. Self-imposed driving limitations are most common among older women [3, 28, 29, 41], with men more likely to continue driving even with higher levels of disability [41]. In the context of longer life expectancies and poorer economic status for older women, premature driving cessation is likely to exacerbate their vulnerability to social isolation [42]. There are mixed findings regarding the effect of living alone on propensity to limit or cease driving. Some reports suggest women living alone may be at greater risk of driving reduction and cessation [28], while others suggest cessation is higher in older women who live with others [29], or that living with another person is predictive of self-regulation rather than cessation [3]. These patterns may in part reflect cohort effects and gender norms where driving has historically been a stronger part of gender identity and life roles for men compared to women. Indeed, data from more recent cohorts indicate higher rates of driving among older women, as well as a narrowing gender gap in driving cessation likelihood [3]. Nevertheless, for older adults faced with involuntary driving cessation, often due to sudden health deterioration, and for whom driving is a strong self-identity, the impact on self-worth and mental health can be devastating. This highlights the need for greater education and preparation for mobility changes in late life.

Longitudinal studies on the impacts of driving cessation indicate older adults typically experience a sudden decrease in out-of-home activities relative to those who continue to drive, followed by a slower trajectory of decline in these activities over the ensuing years [17, 43]. This includes reduced participation in formal and informal volunteering, as well as social engagement and paid employment [17]. There are significant impacts on mental health for those who cease driving. Driving cessation doubles the risk of depressive symptoms in older adults [8]. The capacity to adjust to the sudden mobility restriction and still maintain social participation is dependent on older adults' financial status as well as neighbourhood population density [21, 43]. Financial status impacts both when and how older drivers change driving status. Lower socioeconomic status is associated with higher rates of and earlier cessation [44], and once driving has stopped, more affluent older adults, and those living in higher density urban areas are better able to accommodate for mobility restrictions through access to alternative transport methods [17, 21]. This is also consistent with findings that the risk of social isolation following driving cessation is higher in rural regions [30, 45, 46].

6.6 Characteristics of Older Drivers and Their Driving Behaviour

Certain types of driving errors are more commonly observed among older, experienced drivers as they age. These on-road difficulties are also consistent with the type of crashes that are most common in the age group and can be explained to some extent by age-related changes in cognition and vision. Crash statistics generally reveal that as driver age increases, the crash rate per distance driven also increases, with older drivers being over three times more likely to crash relative to middle-aged drivers [47]. Older drivers tend to be involved in intersection crashes [48], and merging or side-swiping crashes, often due to failure to give way. Similarly, on-road driving assessments and naturalistic driving studies indicate the most common driving errors involve negotiating complex intersections [49], observation, lane keeping, and speed control [38].

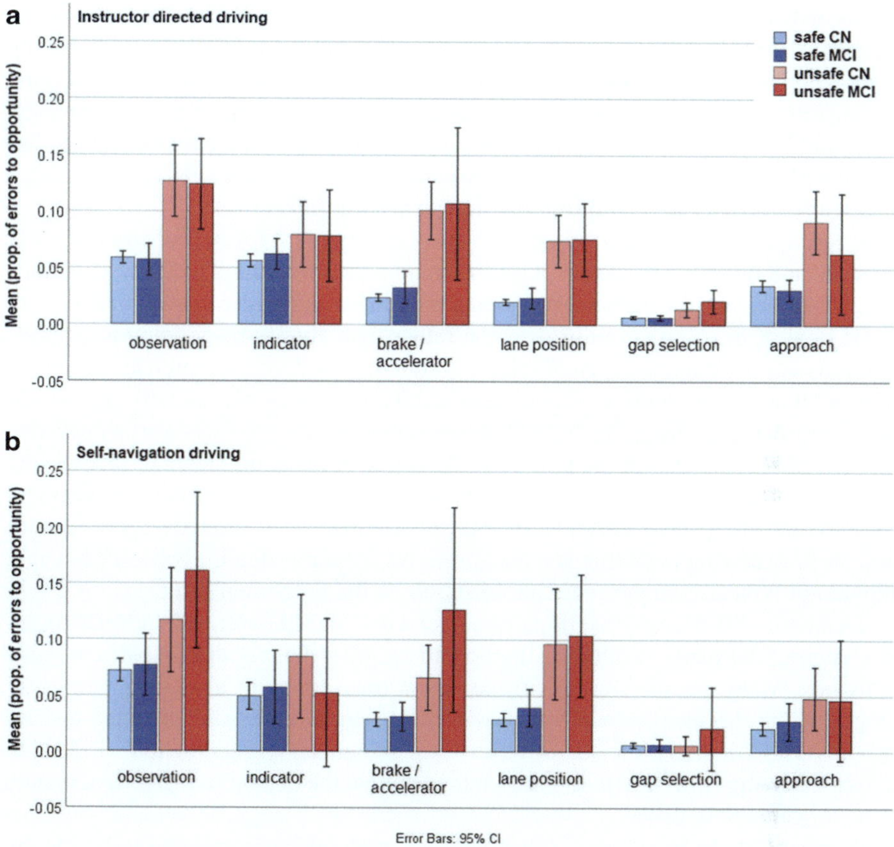

Fig. 6.1 Mean proportion of driving errors committed, relative to opportunity, during a standardised on-road driving assessment by type of error and under (**a**) Instructor directed conditions, and (**b**) Self-navigation conditions. Data are drawn from 296 licensed drivers aged ≥65 years classified by cognitive status and driving safety: cognitively normal (CN) (n = 242, 7% unsafe), and mild cognitive impairment (MCI) (n = 54, 17% unsafe). (Source: [38])

Driving while having to navigate oneself to the destination using road signs tends to increase a driver's cognitive workload, and this often increases error frequency in older drivers when compared to following directions from a passenger (Fig. 6.1).

6.7 Factors Influencing Driving Safety for Older Adults

Chronological age: Safe driving is impacted by several sensory and cognitive abilities which are also vulnerable to declines in normal ageing. In general, there is a slowing of reaction time and processing speed as people age, in addition to declines in executive function and all of these abilities are used in processing information while driving. The overall result of this is that on average older drivers to make more errors on the road, despite their being a range of driving performance. A large observational study of older drivers without dementia showed that all types of driving errors increased with chronological age [6]. These included failures to check blind spots, errors in lane position, errors at give way and stop sign and merging. Importantly, critical errors that raise the risk of a crash also increased with age. The likelihood of making driving errors is associated with the other age-related changes in sensory and cognitive abilities that impact driving safety.

Cognitive ageing: Cognitive abilities that are important for driving are generally speeded and involve processing of information in the visual modality. These include reaction time, and in particular reaction time tasks that are complex and require some type of discrimination or decision rather than simply responding to a single stimulus. Visual scanning, visual selective attention, and visual search are cognitive abilities that interact with declining visual acuity and contrast sensitivity and associated with driving safety [7, 50, 51]. More recently, research has also shown that lower scores on a decision-making task, the Game of Dice, predicted unsafe driving in a large sample of older drivers who undertook an on-road driving assessment [52]. While group level associations are reported between cognitive performance and on-road driving performance, the normative cognitive declines observed in ageing do not typically render older adults unsafe at the individual level.

Dementia, Mild Cognitive Impairment, and driving: In contrast to normal cognitive ageing, dementia results in significant cognitive deficits that impair everyday activities. Many people living with dementia may continue to drive in the early stages of the disease; however, they will need regular assessments as the disease progresses. Ultimately, the cognitive declines associated with dementia will lead to a loss of driving skills and judgement and mean that the person living with dementia is no longer safe to drive.

A recent study examining self-regulation and self-perceptions of driving by adults with early Alzheimer's disease (AD) found that adults with AD and Mild Cognitive Impairment (MCI) reported regulating their driving more than people with normal cognition. They were more likely to rate themselves as excellent drives and expressed less confidence in driving although this study did not evaluate objective driving ability [53].

Mild cognitive impairment is cognitive decline that is measurable, but which does not meet the criteria for dementia. MCI may progress to dementia or remain stable. Research has shown a range of driving abilities in older adults with MCI. While subtle differences in on-road performance are observed at the group level, there is an overlap of distribution of driving across the full range of abilities, with drivers who do not have cognitive impairment. Therefore, having a diagnosis of MCI does not automatically imply an older person has impaired driving [37, 38]. In addition, the widely used screening test for dementia, the Mini-mental State Examination, is not strongly predictive of driving safety [38].

Visual ageing and eye disease: Visual changes in ageing that potentially affect driving are reduction in the useful field of view, reduction in capacity to see in low light condition and at night, reduction in contrast sensitivity, and reduction in motion perception. Population studies show that the prevalence of visual impairment increases from about 1% for adults aged 60–69, to 26% for adults aged 80 and older [54]. However, the typical visual acuity test that is used for licensing is not very sensitive for detecting unsafe older drivers [55].

In addition to the normal age-related changes in visual abilities, age-related eye diseases may increase risk of crashes. The most common eye diseases are cataract, glaucoma [56], and age-related macular degeneration with at least 30% of the older population having a significant cataract in at least one eye [57, 58]. Visual deficits resulting from stroke, such as visual field loss, may also impact driving safety or even lead to driving cessation [59].

Hazard perception: Sensory and cognitive declines may contribute to reduction in the ability to perceive hazards while driving and hazard perception in turn is linked to crash avoidance. Poorer performance on tests of executive function has been linked to poorer hazard perception in adults without dementia or cognitive impairment [60]. Older adults have slower responses to hazards than younger adults [61]. Among older adults, responses to hazards are slower among those with eye disease [62], and older adults are slower to respond in the presence of blur and distractors [63].

6.8 Auditory, Motor, and Postural Control and Driving

In contrast to visual deficits, hearing loss appears to have a lesser impact on driving in later life. A population-based study of 1000 older adults found that adults with either visual or hearing impairment alone, did not have increased crash rates, but that dual sensory loss (vision and hearing impairment) had increased 52% increased risk of a crash [64].

Postural sway which involves the integration of sensorimotor function has also been associated with driving safety [65] as have quadriceps strength, vibration sense, proprioception, neck rotation, and ankle strength [66]. These general abilities may be indicative of overall frailty which is also associated with driving cessation [67]. Adequate muscle strength and neck rotation may also impact the physical management and manoeuvring of a vehicle.

Other factors that contribute to reduced driving safety in the experienced older adult include the quality of driver education, poor driving habits, and de-skilling over time.

6.9 Assessment and Screening to Detect and Manage Unsafe Driving in Later Life

In many regions, health professionals are required to review and assess the impact of an older person's health conditions on their fitness to drive, and act as the first tier in the clinical pathway to licence review and revocation [68–70]. Medical review of conditions that can cause acute deficits, progressive degeneration, fluctuations in levels of alertness, as well as medications are an important part of this. While older adults report that general practitioners are their primary source of information on medical fitness to drive [27], doctors report significant barriers to effective review in terms of training, evidence-based risk assessment tools, and impact on the clinician–patient relationship [71].

Given the increase crash rates among older drivers, and the need to allow unimpaired drivers to keep driving, there is considerable interest in developing methods to detect those who are unsafe, or who would benefit from interventions. While various tests show statistically significant differences between safe and unsafe drivers at the group level, few tests have the sensitivity and specificity to be used in clinical decision-making.

On the whole, research has shown that tests specifically designed to assess driving skills and safety are more effective at identifying unsafe drivers, than neuropsychological tests [72] (Fig. 6.2). Examples of validated off-road screening tests are described below:

The *Useful field of view (UFOV®)* is a computer-based test of visual processing speed and divided attention, demonstrated to predict crash risk [73–77]. *DriveSafe/DriveAware®* [78] is a clinical screening tool for driving safety [40] that requires participants to view each of 15 images of a roundabout and report details about the

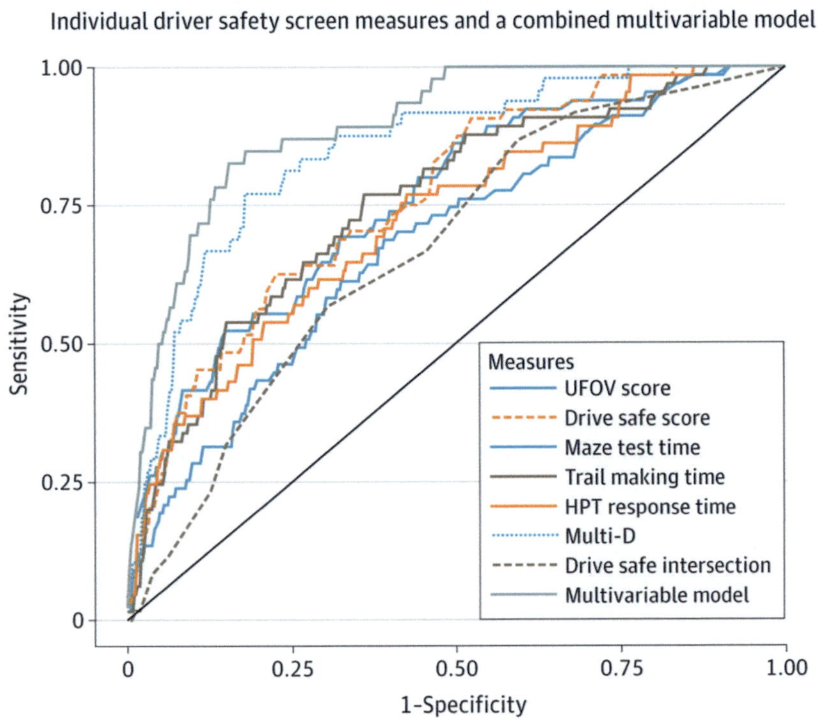

Fig. 6.2 Receiver Operating Characteristic (ROC) Curve showing relative sensitivity and specificity of common off-road brief driver screening measures for discriminating unsafe from safe drivers based on a standardised on-road driver assessment. (Source: [72])

position and direction of travel of pedestrians and vehicle in the image [78]. The *Hazard Perception Test (HPT)* [61] is a computer-based test requiring participants to view videos of traffic scenes and respond via touchscreen when they observed a potential traffic hazard in the video [64]. The *Multi-D* is a computer-based test comprised of three subtests—choice colour reaction time (requiring hand and foot responses and inhibition of responses), a test of sensitivity to central visual motion (using random dot stimuli presented at 3.2 m), and a test of balance or postural sway (using a sway meter to measure body displacement at the level of the waist). The Multi-D subtests have been associated with on-road driving performance [51, 79]. The *OT-DORA Maze test* [80] is a pen-and-paper maze test. Time taken to complete the maze has been associated with driving performance [80, 81].

These tests are often used in conjunction with an on-road driving test conducted by an occupational therapist with specialist training in driver assessment; however, there have been some initiatives that have established a two-step process whereby screening tests are used first in generalised clinics, which then may funnel 'at risk' drivers to receive longer clinical assessments.

Driving simulators may appear to be a promising alternative to on-road driving assessment, but logistical and cost issues have hindered their wide use. A major barrier to their use is that a high proportion of older drivers experience simulator sickness when using simulators [82]. In addition, simulators are expensive to install and do not necessarily correlate highly with on-road experiences.

6.10 Licence Renewal as a Means of Regulation

In Australia and globally, there is variation in whether jurisdictions regulate older drivers, and then for those that do impose regulations, there is further variation in the policies implemented. Some jurisdictions require regular medical clearance from a general practitioner or licence restrictions, others require visual or other screening tests. There is limited research that has compared the different approaches and remains unclear what type of regulation leads to the best outcomes that balance continued driving with identifying unsafe drivers.

In one of the few studies to evaluate driving participation associated with different regulatory requirements, having an age-based testing requirement for renewal of a driver's licence was found to be associated with lower driving rates in older Australians [83]. Further, for people who had the age-based test and those who didn't, the proportion of drivers with probable impairments visually or cognitively were similar.

6.11 Interventions to Improve Driving Safety in Older Adults

In recent years, there has been an increase in focus on improving the skills of older drivers with an increase in agencies offering refresher courses. However, there is still a limited amount of research supporting the efficacy of these programmes. In general, there are five types of interventions. These include (a) classroom-based education which focus on aged-related changes that impact driving and tips on driving and road rules [84, 85]; (b) feedback on driving weaknesses provided by a driving instructor or OT either verbally or using video of real-life driving scenarios [86]; (c) cognitive and skills-based training that focusses on specific areas identified through off-road assessments [87, 88]; (d) driving lessons [85, 89], and (e) training on driving simulators. Some studies have also evaluated combining more than one type of intervention [89–91]. Overall, studies have been limited by small sample sizes and short follow-up intervals. There is also heterogeneity between studies so that it is difficult to combine results of smaller studies.

Despite this, findings from interventions involving cognitive and skills training, and driving lessons, are promising. For example, Anstey et al. (2018) conducted a randomised controlled trial of driving lessons plus feedback ($n = 57$) with follow-up of 6 months [85]. The intervention group improved on their driver rating scale and reduced critical errors at blinded follow-up. Of the intervention group, 64% moved from 'fail' to 'pass' between baseline and follow-up, whereas 24% of the control group improved.

Cognitive training research has found that training on tasks that measure skills required for safe driving may be beneficial. For example, Ball et al. [87] found that training on a speed of processing task using the useful field of view paradigm was associated with reduced crashes. The useful field of view has been associated with driving skills in many studies. Other cognitive training studies have had mixed results, with improvements shown on selected driving skills after training. Further controlled trials targeting driving skills are needed to fully explore the potential of cognitive training to improve driving safety.

Overall while far more research is needed, it appears that providing visual feedback and targeting deficits in the skills known to be important for driving, will provide the most effective interventions for older drivers.

6.12 Summary and Future Directions

Driving in later life remains the main means by which older adults travel and is important for enabling many older people to remain socially engaged. Many older drivers are safe, but age-related changes in cognitive and sensory function impact older drivers' skill and when there is significant impairment, may lead to older drivers being unsafe. Innovations in assistive technology in vehicles have the potential to compensate for some of the age-related changes that affect older drivers. Alongside driving, the benefits of active transport and well-designed public and community transport systems will benefit an ageing population through being environmentally sound and promoting physical activity. Yet driving is expected to remain an integral part of the daily lives of many older adults. Developing the evidence base for assessment of driving safety and designing cars that are adapted for the older person will improve the wellbeing of older drivers.

References

1. Anstey KJ, Li X, Hosking DE, Eramudugolla R. The epidemiology of driving in later life: Sociodemographic, health and functional characteristics, predictors of incident cessation, and driving expectations. Accid Anal Prev. 2017;107:110–6.
2. Babulal GM, Vivoda J, Harmon A, Carr DB, Roe CM, Zikmund-Fisher B. Older adults' expectations about mortality, driving life and years left without driving. J Gerontol Soc Work. 2019;62(8):912–29.
3. Schouten A, Wachs M, Blumenberg EA, King HR. Cohort analysis of driving cessation and limitation among older adults. Transportation. 2022;49(3):841–65.
4. Newbold KB, Scott DM, Spinney JEL, Kanaroglou P, Páez A. Travel behavior within Canada's older *population: a cohort analysis*. J Transp Geogr. 2005;13(4):340–51.
5. BITRE. Australian Infrastructure Statistics—Yearbook 2019. Canberra: ACT; 2019.
6. Anstey KJ, Wood J. Chronological age and age-related cognitive deficits are associated with an increase in multiple types of driving errors in late life. Neuropsychology. 2011;25(5):613.
7. Anstey KJA, Wood J, Lord S, Walker JG. Cognitive, sensory and physical factors enabling driving safety in older adults. Clin Psychol Rev. 2005;25(1):45–65.
8. Chihuri S, Mielenz TJ, DiMaggio CJ, Betz ME, DiGuiseppi C, Jones VC, Li G. Driving cessation and health outcomes in older adults. J Am Geriatr Soc. 2016;64(2):332–41.
9. Leigh-Hunt N, Bagguley D, Bash K, Turner V, Turnbull S, Valtorta N, Caan W. An overview of systematic reviews on the public health consequences of social isolation and loneliness. Public Health. 2017;152:157–71.
10. Hämmig O. Health risks associated with social isolation in general and in young, middle and old age. PLoS One. 2019;14(7):e0219663.
11. Valtorta NK, et al. Loneliness and social isolation as risk factors for coronary heart disease and stroke: systematic review and meta-analysis of longitudinal observational studies. Heart. 2016;102(13):1009–16.
12. Yu B, Steptoe A, Chen Y, Jia X. Social isolation, rather than loneliness, is associated with cognitive decline in older adults: the China Health and Retirement Longitudinal Study. Psychol Med. 2021;51(14):2414–21.
13. Chiao C. Beyond health care: volunteer work, social participation, and late-life general cognitive status in Taiwan. Soc Sci Med. 2019;229:154–60.
14. Evans IEM, Martyr A, Collins R, Brayne C, Clare L. Social isolation and cognitive function in later life: a systematic review and meta-analysis. J Alzheimers Dis. 2019;70(s1):S119–44.
15. Hambisa MT, Dolja-Gore X, Byles JE. Determinants of driving among oldest-old Australian women. J Women Aging. 2022;34(3):351–71.
16. Sallis JF, Bull F, Burdett R, Frank LD, Griffiths P, Giles-Corti B, Stevenson M. Use of science to guide city planning policy and practice: how to achieve healthy and sustainable future cities. Lancet. 2016;388(10062):2936–47.
17. Curl AL, Stowe JD, Cooney TM, Proulx CM. Giving up the keys: how driving cessation affects engagement in later life. Gerontologist. 2014;54(3):423–33.
18. Steptoe A, Fancourt D. Leading a meaningful life at older ages and its relationship with social engagement, prosperity, health, biology, and time use. Proc Natl Acad Sci. 2019;116(4):1207–12.
19. Jiang D, Hosking D, Burns R, Anstey KJ. Volunteering benefits life satisfaction over 4 years: the moderating role of social network size. Aust J Psychol. 2019;71(2):183–92.
20. Jenkinson CE, Dickens AP, Jones K, Thompson-Coon J, Taylor RS, Rogers M, Bambra CL, Lang I, Richards SH. Is volunteering a public health intervention? A systematic review and meta-analysis of the health and survival of volunteers. BMC Public Health. 2013;13:773.
21. Phillips CB, Freed SA, Ross LA. Older adult lifespace varies by driving status and residential population density. Transp Res Rec. 2019;2673(7):586–95.

22. Tran Y, Hashimoto N, Ando T, Sato T, Konishi N, Takeda Y, Akamatsu M. Associations between motorized transport access, out-of-home activities, and life-space mobility in older adults in Japan. BMC Public Health. 2022;22(1):676.
23. Douma L, Steverink N, Meijering L. Geographical life-space and subjective wellbeing in later life. Health Place. 2021;70:102608.
24. Kennedy RE, Sawyer P, Williams CP, Lo AX, Ritchie CS, Roth DL, Allman RM, Brown CJ. Life-space mobility change predicts 6-month mortality. J Am Geriatr Soc. 2017;65(4):833–8.
25. Kamioka Y, Miura Y, Matsuda T, Iijima Y, Suzuki A, Nakazato K, Saito H, Arita M. Changes in social participation and life-space mobility in newly enrolled home-based rehabilitation users over 6 months. J Phys Ther Sci. 2020;32(6):375–84.
26. Mazer B, Chen Y-T, Vrkljan B, Marshall SC, Charlton JL, Koppel S, et al. Comparison of older and middle-aged drivers' driving performance in a naturalistic setting. Accid Anal Prev. 2021;161:106343.
27. Sargent-Cox KA, Windsor T, Walker J, Anstey KJ. Health literacy of older drivers and the importance of health experience for self-regulation of driving behaviour. Accid Anal Prev. 2011;43(3):898–905.
28. Ang BH, Oxley JA, Chen WS, Yap KK, Song KP, Lee SWH. To reduce or to cease: a systematic review and meta-analysis of quantitative studies on self-regulation of driving. J Saf Res. 2019;70:243–51.
29. Anstey KJ, Windsor TD, Luszcz MA, Andrews GR. Predicting driving cessation over 5 years in older adults: psychological well-being and cognitive competence are stronger predictors than physical health. J Am Geriatr Soc. 2006;54(1):121–6.
30. Hambisa MT, Dolja-Gore X, Byles JE. Predictors of driving among older Australian women from 2002 to 2011: a longitudinal analysis of Australian Longitudinal Study on Women's Health based on the World Health Organization's Healthy Ageing Framework. J Transp Health. 2021;22:101116.
31. Wood JM, Black AA. Ocular disease and driving. Clin Exp Optom. 2016;99(5):395–401.
32. Agramunt S, Meuleners LB, Fraser ML, Chow KC, Ng JQ, Raja V. First and second eye cataract surgery and driver self-regulation among older drivers with bilateral cataract: a prospective cohort study. BMC Geriatr. 2018;18(1):1–8.
33. Fraser ML, Meuleners LB, Ng JQ, Morlet N. Driver self-regulation and depressive symptoms in cataract patients awaiting surgery: a cross-sectional study. BMC Ophthalmol. 2013;13:45.
34. White J, Hambisa MT, Cavenagh D, Dolja-Gore X, Byles J. Understanding the relationship between eye disease and driving in very old Australian women: a longitudinal thematic evaluation. BMC Ophthalmol. 2022;22(1):277.
35. Doi T, Tsutsumimoto K, Ishii H, Nakakubo S, Kurita S, Shimada H. Frailty and driving status associated with disability: a 24-month follow-up longitudinal study. BMJ Open. 2021;11(4):e042468.
36. Feng YR, Meuleners L, Stevenson M, Heyworth J, Murray K, Fraser M, Maher S. A longitudinal study examining self-regulation practices in older drivers with and without suspected mild cognitive impairment. Clin Interv Aging. 2021;16:2069–78.
37. Anstey KJ, Eramudugolla R, Chopra S, Price J, Wood JM. Assessment of driving safety in older adults with mild cognitive impairment. J Alzheimers Dis. 2017;57(4):1197–205.
38. Eramudugolla R, Huque MH, Wood J, Anstey KJ. On-road behavior in older drivers with mild cognitive impairment. J Am Med Dir Assoc. 2021;22(2):399–405.
39. Wood JM, Lacherez PF, Anstey KJ. Not all older adults have insight into their driving abilities: evidence from an on-road assessment and implications for policy. J Gerontol A Biol Sci Med Sci. 2013;68(5):559–66.
40. Horswill MS, Anstey KJ, Hatherly C, Wood JM, Pachana NA. Older drivers' insight into their hazard perception ability. Accid Anal Prev. 2011;43(6):2121–7.
41. Ross LA, Anstey KJ, Kiely KM, Windsor TD, Byles JE, Luszcz MA, Mitchell P. Older drivers in Australia: trends in driving status and cognitive and visual impairment. J Am Geriatr Soc. 2009;57(10):1868–73.

42. Byles JE, Leigh L, Vo K, Forder P, Curryer C. Life space and mental health: a study of older community-dwelling persons in Australia. Aging Ment Health. 2015;19(2):98–106.
43. Huisingh C, Levitan EB, Sawyer P, Kennedy R, Brown CJ, McGwin G. Impact of driving cessation on trajectories of life-space scores among community-dwelling older adults. J Appl Gerontol. 2017;36(12):1433–52.
44. Vivoda JM, Walker RM, Cao J, Koumoutzis A. How accumulated wealth affects driving reduction and cessation. Gerontologist. 2020;60(7):1273–81.
45. Strogatz D, Mielenz TJ, Johnson AK, Baker IR, Robinson M, Mebust SP, Andrews HF, Betz ME, Eby DW, Johnson RM, Jones VC, Leu CS, Molnar LJ, Rebok GW, Li G. Importance of driving and potential impact of driving cessation for rural and urban older adults. J Rural Health. 2020;36(1):88–93.
46. Lynch L, Mielenz TJ, Li G, Eby DW, Molnar LJ, Betz ME, DiGuiseppi C, Hill LL, Jones V, Strogatz D. Rate of social isolation by geographic location among older adults: AAA LongROAD Study. Front Public Health. 2021;9:791683.
47. Pitta LSR, Quintas JL, Trindade IOA, Belchior P, Gameiro KDSD, Gomes CM, Nóbrega OT, Camargos EF. Older drivers are at increased risk of fatal crash involvement: results of a systematic review and meta-analysis. Arch Gerontol Geriatr. 2021;95:104414.48.
48. Swain TA, McGwin G Jr, Antin JF, Wood JM, Owsley C. Left turns by older drivers with vision impairment: a naturalistic driving study. Innov Aging. 2021;5(3):igab026.
49. Seacrist T, Douglas EC, Hannan C, Rogers R, Belwadi A, Loeb H. Near crash characteristics among risky drivers using the SHRP2 naturalistic driving study. J Saf Res. 2020;73:263–9.
50. Wood JM, Troutbeck R. Effect of visual impairment on driving. Hum Factors. 1994;36(3):476–87.
51. Anstey KJ, Horswill MS, Wood JM, Hatherly C. The role of cognitive and visual abilities as predictors in the Multifactorial Model of Driving Safety. Accid Anal Prev. 2012;45:766–74.
52. Brady B, Eramudugolla R, Wood JM, Anstey KJ. Association between decision-making under risk conditions and on-road driving safety among older drivers. Neuropsychology. 2021;35(6):622–9.
53. Davis R, Owens M. Self-regulation of driving behaviors in persons with early-stage Alzheimer's disease. J Gerontol Nurs. 2021;47(1):21–7.
54. Wang JJ, Foran S, Mitchell P. Age-specific prevalence and causes of bilateral and unilateral visual impairment in older Australians: the Blue Mountains Eye Study. Clin Exp Ophthalmol. 2000;28(4):268–73.
55. Eramudugolla R, Laird M, Black AA, Cameron ID, Wood JM, Anstey KJ. Inability of the Mini-Mental State Exam (MMSE) and high-contrast visual acuity to identify unsafe drivers. Accid Anal Prev. 2022;168:106595.
56. Blane A. Through the looking glass: a review of the literature investigating the impact of glaucoma on crash risk, driving performance, and driver self-regulation in older drivers. J Glaucoma. 2016;25(1):113–21.
57. Mitchell P, Cumming RG, Attebo K, Panchapakesan J. Prevalence of cataract in Australia: the Blue Mountains eye study. Ophthalmology. 1997;104(4):581–8.
58. Rochtchina E, Mukesh BN, Wang JJ, McCarty CA, Taylor HR, Mitchell P. Projected prevalence of age-related cataract and cataract surgery in Australia for the years 2001 and 2021: pooled data from two population-based surveys. Clin Exp Ophthalmol. 2003;31(3):233–6.
59. Bro T, Andersson J. The effects of visual field loss from stroke on performance in a driving simulator. Optom Vis Sci. 2022;99(9):679–86.
60. McInerney K, Suhr J. Neuropsychological correlates of hazard perception in older adults. J Int Neuropsychol Soc. 2016;22(3):332–40.
61. Horswill MS, Anstey KJ, Hatherly CG, Wood JM. The crash involvement of older drivers is associated with their hazard perception latencies. J Int Neuropsychol Soc. 2010;16(5):939–44.
62. Wood JM, Black AA, Anstey KJ, Horswill MS. Hazard perception in older drivers with eye disease. Transl Vis Sci Technol. 2021;10(1):31.

63. Green KA, McGwin G Jr, Owsley C. Associations between visual, hearing, and dual sensory impairments and history of motor vehicle collision involvement of older drivers. J Am Geriatr Soc. 2013;61(2):252–7.
64. Wood JM, Anstey KJ, Kerr GK, Lacherez PF, Lord S. A multidomain approach for predicting older driver safety under in-traffic road conditions. J Am Geriatr Soc. 2008;56(6):986–93.
65. Lacherez P, Wood JM, Anstey KJ, Lord SR. Sensorimotor and postural control factors associated with driving safety in a community-dwelling older driver population. J Gerontol A Biol Sci Med Sci. 2014;69(2):240–4.
66. Ishii H, Doi T, Tsutsumimoto K, Nakakubo S, Kurita S, Shimada H. Driving cessation and physical frailty in community-dwelling older adults: a longitudinal study. Geriatr Gerontol Int. 2021;21(11):1047–52.
67. Austroads. Assessing Fitness to Drive. 2022 Sydney, Australia. https://austroads.com.au/drivers-and-vehicles/assessing-fitness-to-drive. Accessed 8 Feb 2023.
68. CMA driver's guide : determining medical fitness to operate motor vehicles. – 10th edition, ISBN 978-1-897490-56-3. 2015. https://driversguide.ca/.
69. American Medical Association. Physician's guide to assessing and counseling older drivers. Chicago: American Medical Association; 2010.
70. McKsernan E, Chia SYD, Traynor V, Veerhuis N, McNeil K, Pond CD. Driving assessments for older adult patients: interviews with general practitioners to gauge current strategies and future directions. Aust J Gen Pract. 2022;51(6):457–62.
71. Anstey KJ, Eramudugolla R, Huque MH, Horswill M, Kiely K, Black A, Wood J. Validation of brief screening tools to identify impaired driving among older adults in Australia. JAMA Netw Open. 2020;3(6):e208263.
72. Owsley C, Ball K, McGwin G Jr, Sloane ME, Roenker DL, White MF, Overley ET. Visual processing impairment and risk of motor vehicle crash among older adults. JAMA. 1998;279(14):1083–8.
73. Ball KK, Roenker DL, Wadley VG, Edwards JD, Roth DL, McGwin G Jr, Raleigh R, Joyce JJ, Cissell GM, Dube T. Can high-risk older drivers be identified through performance-based measures in a Department of Motor Vehicles setting? J Am Geriatr Soc. 2006;54(1):77–84.
74. Ball K, Owsley C. The useful field of view test: a new technique for evaluating age-related declines in visual function. J Am Optom Assoc. 1993;64(1):71–9.
75. Edwards JD, Ross LA, Wadley VG, Clay OJ, Crowe M, Roenker DL, Ball KK. The useful field of view test: normative data for older adults. Arch Clin Neuropsychol. 2006;21(4):275–86.
76. Myers RS, Ball KK, Kalina TD, Roth DL, Goode KT. Relation of useful field of view and other screening tests to on-road driving performance. Percept Mot Skills. 2000;91(1):279–90.
77. Kay LG, Bundy AC, Clemson LM. Predicting fitness to drive using the visual recognition slide test (USyd). Am J Occup Ther. 2008;62(2):187–97.
78. Kay LG, Bundy AC, Clemson LM. Predicting fitness to drive in people with cognitive impairments by using DriveSafe and DriveAware. Arch Phys Med Rehabil. 2009;90(9):1514–22.
79. Krishnasamy C, Unsworth C. Validity of the occupational therapy-drive home Maze Test for right and left handed test takers. Accid Anal Prev. 2012;49:274–7.
80. Staplin L, Gish KW, Lococo KH, Joyce JJ, Sifrit KJ. The Maze Test: a significant predictor of older driver crash risk. Accid Anal Prev. 2013;50:483–9.
81. Dużmańska N, Strojny P, Strojny A. Can simulator sickness be avoided? A review on temporal aspects of simulator sickness. Front Psychol. 2018;9:2132.
82. Ross LA, Browning C, Luszcz MA, Mitchell P, Anstey KJ. Age-based testing for driver's license renewal: potential implications for older Australians. J Am Geriatr Soc. 2011;59(2):281–5.
83. Bédard M, Isherwood I, Moore E, Gibbons C, Lindstrom W. Evaluation of a re-training program for older drivers. Can J Public Health. 2004;95(4):295–8.
84. Anstey KJ, Eramudugolla R, Kiely KM, Price J. Effect of tailored on-road driving lessons on driving safety in older adults: a randomised controlled trial. Accid Anal Prev. 2018;115:1–10.
85. Lavallière M, Simoneau M, Tremblay M, Laurendeau D, Teasdale N. Active training and driving-specific feedback improve older drivers' visual search prior to lane changes. BMC Geriatr. 2012;12(1):1–9.

86. Ball K, Edwards JD, Ross LA, McGwin G Jr. Cognitive training decreases motor vehicle collision involvement of older drivers. J Am Geriatr Soc. 2010;58(11):2107–13.
87. Eramudugolla R, Kiely KM, Chopra S, Anstey KJ. Effect of speed of processing training on older driver screening measures. Front Aging Neurosci. 2017;9:338.
88. Mullen NW, et al. Older driver performance on a simulator: associations between simulated tasks and cognition. Adv Transp Stud. 2008. Special Issue. 31–42.
89. Roenker DL, Cissell GM, Ball KK, Wadley VG, Edwards JD. Speed-of-processing and driving simulator training result in improved driving performance. Hum factors. 2003;45(2):218–33.
90. Sawula E, Polgar J, Porter MM, Gagnon S, Weaver B, Nakagawa S, et al. The combined effects of on-road and simulator training with feedback on older drivers' on-road performance: Evidence from a randomized controlled trial. Traffic injury prevention. 2018;19(3):241–49.
91. Bedard M, et al. The combination of two training approaches to improve older adults' driving safety. Traffic Inj Prev. 2008;9(1):70–6.
92. Lee SS, et al. Eye movements and road hazard detection: effects of blur and distractors. Optom Vis Sci. 2016;93(9): 1137–46.

Creative Ageing

7

Jane W. Davidson

7.1 Introduction

Finding appropriate and innovative psychosocial structures to support increased longevity is a priority for all: individuals, families and communities, local, state, and federal government services, public and private sector employment, and national economies.

Creative Ageing, broadly conceived, describes an idea that focuses on exploring the creativity of older adults using meaningful participatory engagement to stimulate these individuals and their communities and prepare them to manage old age. It can include challenging stereotypes of older people and offer pleasure, social and cultural engagement. Aligned with gerontological constructs of healthy ageing and successful ageing that emerged in the 1960s, creative ageing is a term that began circulation in the 1970s. Programmes have been developed and run in North America, Europe, and Australasia, some of which have been supported by government agencies. The spectrum of creative engagements has embraced activities such as gardening and cooking, but the primary locus of the approach has been creative arts activities. As the decades have progressed, creative arts activities have been shown to offer an approach to ameliorating the challenges associated with ageing that is more meaningful and less costly than pharmacological alternatives. Research evidence has revealed that protective and even restorative impact on cognitive and physical wellbeing and brain health can be attained. The current chapter offers an overview of how Creative Ageing emerged, and what it comprises in the current global context. A summary of the types of activities and outcomes achieved is given, alongside an exploration of

J. W. Davidson (✉)
Faculty of Fine Arts and Music, University of Melbourne, Melbourne, VIC, Australia
e-mail: j.davidson@unimelb.edu.au

J. Byles (ed.), *What Matters for Healthy Ageing*, Topics in Geriatric Care,
https://doi.org/10.1007/978-981-96-0462-3_7

how Creative Ageing programmes and their implementation can be developed for further outcomes.

7.2 The Concept of Creative Ageing

'Creative Ageing' is a policy idea emergent in Western cultures that involves creative activities that engage older participants intellectually, physically, emotionally and socially, and are regarded as offering a range of benefits that result in improved health and wellbeing [1–3]. The activities provide opportunities to express and understand lived experience and are acknowledged as being important to personal and cultural identity. The range of creative ageing activities typically focuses on the arts, including performing arts, visual arts, creative writing, or digital technologies [4].

A general history of the Creative Ageing Movement has been traced by Klimczuk [5], noting the importance of work developed in the 1960s drawing on theoretical frameworks emerging in gerontology such as 'active aging', 'quality of life', 'healthy aging', and 'mental capital' [6, 7]. These approaches typically explore the navigation of 'life challenges' such as coping with physical restriction or decline associated with ageing and/or the increased experience of grief and loss through bereavement. They also engage with 'resources' that may be gained from some forms of material support or socio-cultural interactions to aid in managing these challenging circumstances and conditions.

Applying these ideas to arts programmes, in the 1970s American artists like Susan Perlstein (founder of Elders Share the Arts) and Liz Lerman (creator of the Dance Exchange) began lobbying for policies to support their work [8]. By the 1990s, through bodies such as the Society for the Arts in Healthcare founded in the USA and the work of Gulbenkian Calouste Foundation in the UK, these types of arts activities became closely associated with the community arts movement. In Europe, varieties of activities were organised through the Universities of the Third Age movement, with many courses and workshops [5, 9]. The UK Parliament [10] and USA groups (e.g. American for the Arts National Conventions and Arts Policy Roundtables, 2022) [11], are now beginning to gain traction nationally with policy initiatives, and Australians are also receiving more direct governmental acknowledgement and support for the broader field of arts and health (e.g. the recent new Cultural Policy, Revive, 2023 [12]; and the Australia Council for the Arts Report, 2022) [13]. The overall movement is often associated with advertising slogans such as 'sing for health' or 'arts for wellbeing.' The concept of using 'arts on prescription' in which local community medical centres refer individuals to an arts activity rather than prescribing a pharmacological treatment is also growing as a global social movement [14].

Gene D. Cohen, a gerontological psychiatrist, has been regarded as a key intellectual figure in the development of the creative ageing concept. Cohen proposed that the way in which a person manifests their neurological, emotional, intellectual, and psychological capacities expands across the life course due to an inner drive which occurs through a series of human potential phases that ‘reflect evolving mental maturity, ongoing human development, and psychological growth as we age’ [15, p. 7]. Arguing that wisdom and creativity emerge particularly from mid to later life, Cohen asserts that creativity has a central role in relationship building and management, and in responding to challenges with novel directions and solutions. Rejecting stereotypical theories of disengagement in later life, he designed a support tool which he labelled the ‘Social Portfolio’. Guided by the tool, an individual lists vital activities along dimensions that account for different potential contexts, such as of low to high mobility, solo to group pursuits, periods of great loss, or experiencing disability.

Cohen undertook ‘The Creativity and Ageing Study’ [16] involving 300 people aged 65 and older (mean = 80 years) who were living independently and engaged in a weekly participatory arts programme, involving between-session assignments and outings to exhibitions and concerts. It was an important piece of research not least because an equal number of participants took part in their routine activities, thus meaning that the impact of arts engagements could be compared in a controlled trail. Measures assessed mental health, physical health, and social functioning. One year after baseline measurement, the control group reported declining health and increased medication whereas the arts groups reported statistically fewer doctor visits than the control group and took fewer medications after the study. Mental health was also positively affected, and those who took part in arts groups were more inclined to take up new additional activities than the controls. However, this landmark study was not fully analysed, and only the impacts of group singing were published in a peer-reviewed journal. Despite these flaws, it has become acknowledged as a significant moment in the field, and Cohen did much to promote the importance of this type of study [17]. The work demonstrated the potential of creative arts engagements to offer the ageing person physical, cognitive, and social expansion and growth.

Another important body of work that usefully sits within a Creative Ageing approach comes from educational psychology, developed through work on the Music for Life project across the period 2010–2014 [18, 19]. In this project, the basic psychological needs theory of Deci and Ryan [20] was adapted and through extensive investigative study of 500 older people revealed that three factors underpinned positive outcomes through artistic engagement (in their case, music): sense of purpose and positive outlook; self-perceptions of autonomy and control; and social relationships, competence, and recognised accomplishment. This work showed that artistic engagement fostered growth in all these aspects for those who engaged positively. The approach has been extended in other studies including Lee et al. [21]. As this chapter unfurls, evidence will highlight how opportunities that stimulate the creativity of older people support psychological needs and engender a range of positive cognitive and physical outcomes.

The current Creative Ageing movement did not emerge in a vacuum, indeed associations between arts and wellbeing have been reported for as long as records have been kept. More than 4000 years ago, flute music was prescribed in China to calm an over-excited foetus and there is evidence that ancient Egyptians used arts for a range of therapeutic purposes at least as early as 1500 BC. The Classical Greek philosophers including Plato (427–347 BCE) and Aristotle (384–322 BCE) also proposed arts activities to calm mood [22]. Australian Aboriginal culture is the oldest continuous culture in existence, with artistic practices being central to knowledge formation, meaning, and belief. For example, the concept of the Dreamtime offers an account of how peoples came to inhabit various places, by being sung into existence [23]. 'Songlines' offer a link between collective memory and associations of place and environment and traces of songlines are recorded in songs, stories, dance, and painting. A person finds their way across the land by singing the right sequence of songs, which describe the location of landmarks, waterholes, and other natural phenomena. In this cultural framework, the continent has a system of songlines, describing land over which the song passes. Traditional Aboriginal people regard all land as sacred, and the songs keep the land 'alive'. Thus, in this cultural context, arts activities have vital social and ecological roles and to be an older Aboriginal person means that engagement in artistic practices is a vital part of lived experience for wellbeing outcomes [24, 25]. Of further relevance to this chapter, in many First Nations cultures, an elder is a member of a community who has gained recognition as a custodian of cultural knowledge and lore. Elders have permission to disclose knowledge related to culture and its practices. There is a strong and positive association between ageing, wisdom, wellbeing, and arts and cultural practice [26].

Looking to understand and work within cultural practices and beliefs is certainly an important consideration as Creative Ageing develops as a concept, a field of research, and a social care practice. For many, lived experience does not include regular artistic experiences and the value of older people is often disregarded, so when aiming to bring benefit and change, barriers can be difficult to overcome. Ongoing dialogue between communities, culture groups, facilitators, professional associations, and governmental agencies is necessary to both develop and optimise creative quality life experiences for older people, especially if comprehensive and inclusive offerings are to be created. As the Creative Ageing approach expands, more collaboration between key stakeholders will certainly aid in understanding why and how the arts can work to bring a range of psychosocial benefits to older people.

7.3 The Existing Body of Evidence

The field of Creative Ageing is amassing a body of arts-based evidence that reveals the positive impact of arts with older people. From the onset, it is important to note that studies have tended to be restricted to Western-arts contexts and have been much more focused on some forms of activity over others. Some of these existing studies are now discussed, focusing first on social networks and self-concept, then cognitive impact, and concluding with a specific focus on people living with dementia.

7.3.1 Social Networking Benefits of Creative Arts Engagement with Older People

Research reveals that arts engagements can increase opportunity for interpersonal relationships and practical and emotional support. The activities promote cooperative group work with an emphasis on enhancing social cohesion. Indeed, in both nursing homes and community settings, arts have been shown to increase socialisation and social interaction (see reviews in Steen et al. [27], Curtis et al. [28]). Further to this, by engaging with creative design thinking we can shape residential spaces to facilitate the social dynamics of those living in them [29]. Liddle et al. [30] explored older women's art and craft participation, concluding that 'participation in art and craft activities [can create] a symbolic wholeness, where it is possible to complete items, help others, be valued and enjoy the moment' [30, p. 337]. Maidment and McFarlane [31] also investigated crafting, highlighting the importance of belonging to the craft group for closeness, learning, new social networks, and engendering self-agency.

A study comparing weekly participation in newly formed singing groups with participation in crafts and creative writing groups collected data focused on determining levels of social connection between group members at months 1, 3, and 7. All groups were facilitated by professional and experienced tutors. The results showed that by month 7, all participants felt equally connected, but the singers reported significantly higher levels of social closeness at time 1. These results are framed in terms of the affect elicited by the singing activity generating an 'ice-breaker' effect for social bonding [32].

Theoretical accounts of empirical results inevitably vary, though the closeness achieved in singing groups is additionally reported in longitudinal qualitative work with singing groups [33–35]. In this work, participants spoke about a range of social benefits, but observed that they felt 'acceptance', 'fellowship', 'as if in a family or at home' and 'safe'. One member, a widow who had migrated to a new country in her 80s to move close to her daughter, noted that making social connections was 'quick' through the singing, and another member referred specifically to singing as being able to 'break down barriers'. The older participants were also incredibly aware of the social processes affecting them. Proximity and physical touch were experiences that could be observed within the singing group in a manner that may not occur in other social contexts. One woman noted that after her husband died, she did not experience physical proximity to others anymore. However, being in the singing group it was far easier to achieve closer contact with people, something she believed was owing to the music itself. Indeed, several singers referred to the experience of being surrounded by the sound, enveloped by it.

The evidence suggests therefore that the social networking achieved in arts activities can result in social wellbeing benefit, including sense of affirmation and bonding. The evidence also indicates that some arts activities may be more appropriate for specific outcomes.

7.3.2 Self-Worth, Sense of Purpose, Achievement, and Countering Loneliness

The development of self-worth is another strong potential outcome of arts engagements for older people. Evidence suggests that through creativity and/or challenges associated with artistic activity, a stronger sense of sense of self is facilitated which in turn affirms identity and so improves self-esteem [36, 37]. Whether performing at high levels or simply 'for the fun of it', research shows that these engagements can lead to feelings of both pride and satisfaction. Indeed, several studies have highlighted how exhibiting, presenting, or performing an artwork can not only improve self-esteem, but also generate a sense of offering value and giving to others. For example, Southcott [38] and Davidson [33] both found that older people enjoyed performing to others in care homes, at seniors' festivals and alike for these reasons.

Engaging in a creative arts group activity can also reduce feelings of loneliness for older people, especially those living alone. One study explored receptive arts, that is, visits to the cinema, museums, galleries, exhibitions, theatre, concerts, or opera [39, 40]. Data were collected by English Longitudinal Study of Ageing (ELSA) and the authors explored responses from waves 2 (2004–2005) and 7 (2014–2015) examining cross-sectional (n = 6222) and longitudinal (n = 3127) associations between the numbers and frequency of receptive arts engagement and loneliness (drawing on results from the three-item short form of the Revised UCLA Loneliness Scale). Adjusting for sociodemographic, economic, health and social, community and civic engagement factors, the results showed negative associations between engagement with any of the receptive arts activities and experiences of loneliness.

The advantage of the ELSA study is that it could draw on population-based data to capture responses from thousands, rather than the typically small-scale studies in arts fields, and it does show clear value in arts engagements in terms of addressing perceived loneliness. However, the work did have several limitations which are common to much work across the entire field of study. For example, the sample was generally educated, healthier, and more socially engaged than the population at large. Further to this, those who were reporting loneliness tended not to engage with the types of arts engagements listed in ELSA and so were missed from the study.

Todd et al. [41] reported on a series of museum programmes that recruited participants sampled across age, ethnicity, previous museum attendance, educational attainment, mobility levels, and most recent healthcare visits. These individuals were aged 65–94 and self-identified as being lonely or socially isolated, and they typically lived alone and did not regularly attend other clubs or societies. In the study, they took part in activities including object handling, participatory arts, and singing. The results showed that participants perceived a reduction in loneliness and that the arts practices took place in a context perceived to be safe and stimulating, offering positive experiences which led to enhanced self-esteem [41].

Another study of creative craft activities explored the feelings of self-worth and positive emotions for older female participants in rural art and craft groups who worked on flower arranging, self-portraits using iPads, origami, canvas bag making, glass jar and terracotta plant pot painting, and 3D wooden model making [42]. These participants spoke at length about the value they experienced in the art and craft activities, noting the emotional synchrony they felt with others, and how the activities also bolstered self-worth and sense of achievement as well as offering participants control and autonomy in their approach to the artwork being undertaken. This study also involved the older participants in artistic co-production, which was critical to their experience and the sense of investment.

Another important insight to self-identity and artistic expression is found in a study of Icelandic men singing both in a male voice choir and purposefully in their daily lives, for example, singing with grandchildren, or when in the farm shed [43]. The work is both an ethnography of the men and an autoethnography of the conductor, researcher (Faulkner) which traces experiences to underscore how basic psychological needs are addressed and met (see [18]), and how personal meaning, self-concept, and identity are created and played out in musical interactions. This work neatly ties back to the strong value of culture and the relationship to context (nature, the environment, spirituality/beliefs) that arts activities embedded in historical cultural practices support (see earlier for references to Australian Aboriginal and other First Nations arts practices).

In addition to social networking, inclusion, affirmation and development of self-worth, purpose, control and autonomy, the work undertaken in the Creative Ageing Movement has also been able to address cognitive and physical challenges that are often associated with the process of ageing.

7.3.3 Impact of Creative Arts on Older People's Cognitive and Physical Skills

Studies linked to musical expertise acquired prior to entering older age have shown that lasting cognitive and physical benefits are likely to be experienced. For example, it has been reported that older musicians out-perform non-musicians on a range of executive functions including planning, fluency, and inhibition [44]. These types of behavioural differences have been shown at the neural level [45]. Other cognitive tasks where older musicians showed superior performance over non-musicians included long-term memory [46], working memory and visuospatial processing [47] and speech perception [48]. Hanna-Plady and MacKay [49] collected biographical data relating to older musicians and administered a series of cognitive tests to discover that transfer effects to general cognitive processes occurred. Also, in a study of the Scottish Lothian Birth Cohort of 1936, Okely et al. [50] tested whether experience of playing a musical instrument in childhood affected cognitive ability in later life. Participants had completed general cognitive-ability assessments at ages 11 and 70 and reported their lifetime experience of playing a musical instrument at age 82. Positive association between playing a musical instrument and change in general cognitive ability between ages 11 and 70 was found. The more musically experienced were likely to show gains in general cognitive ability.

These results again indicate that playing a musical instrument offers a long-term cognitive advantage.

The results above need to be considered in the context of factors such as age when musical training began, level of expertise, and amount of formal training and current practice in older age, which may all have specific influences on cognition [51]. Also, without detailed real-time data it is hard to ascertain actual amounts of work undertaken and what changes occurred across a life course. While these elements need more expansive study, short-term changes have been traced in detail. For example, when older people aged between 60 and 85 were offered 30 min of instrumental lessons and were asked to undertake 3 h of practice a week, after 6 months of learning they were found to have significantly improve performance on cognitive tests, motor skills, executive functions, and working memory, when compared to a non-active control group [52].

Arts activities other than music can improve cognitive functioning, memory, and executive function. Indeed, a lengthy scoping review by Fancourt and Finn [53] explores these aspects in detail. For example, dance classes can improve memory, learning, and attention (see work by Lazarou et al. [54] and Zhao et al. [55]) partly through enhancing motor learning [56]. Additionally, theatre engagements in community settings and in retirement homes have been shown to improve memory and executive function [57], and visual art training has improved auditory evoked responses to sounds and visual processing [58]. Also, going to museums, galleries, the theatre, concerts, or the opera at least once every few months in older age has been associated with a slower rate of cognitive decline and a lower risk of developing dementia [59, 60].

Reduction in brain volume is frequently associated with ageing, mainly impacting the pre-frontal cortex, and thus influencing working memory and executive function. In grey matter, cortical volume decreases as a result of age-related shrinking of cells and reduced synaptic density and in white matter, axonal deflection produces defective neuronal transmission. However, decrease in volume is not inevitable. A study comparing dance and exercise programmes with 63–80-year-olds offers compelling results [59]. Participants were randomly assigned to twice-weekly 90-min dance or a standard fitness training programme for a period of 6 months. Results revealed that both interventions showed a comparable increase in physical fitness, and cognitive improvements in attention and spatial memory. However, the blood results showed an increase in plasma in the dancers and there were significant differences in brain volumes, with the dancing producing larger volume increases in cingulate cortex, insula, corpus callosum, and sensorimotor cortex. The authors suggested that more cognitive changes may emerge after the structural changes have occurred, but they did not take further cognitive measures. Nonetheless, this study indicated with some compelling evidence that dance may counteract brain shrinkage associated with ageing [61].

7.3.4 Impact of Creative Arts on those Experiencing Dementia

Several studies reveal benefits from listening to and making music, resulting in improved cognition, speech improvements including verbal fluency, and visuospatial skills (see Fusar-Poli et al. [62] and Fancourt and Finn [53, 59, 60]. In fact, singing offers many positive outcomes on a range of cognitive skills relating to attention, memory, and executive function [63]. Dance movement therapy and music have also been found to support embodied nonverbal communication [64]. Literature activities (e.g. group reading or storytelling) positively affect memory, listening, attention, and conversation skills [65].

Responding to a significant increase in governmental support for health using arts, a pre- and post-test study was conducted in the Netherlands using a mixed-method design to explore how art activities influence the wellbeing of long-term dementia care residents and older people with chronic psychiatric disorders [66]. Care residents took part in either (a) dance, (b) music and movement, or (c) visual arts, the activities being co-created with the residents and executed by artists and caregivers together in 8 to 10 weeks. Data were collected via group discussions with artists, caregivers, and residents. In increasing social opportunity, the results indicated that participating in an art activity positively increased relationships, and consequently, also improved self-esteem; in other words, those living with dementia responded in ways similar to other older people described in other studies mentioned earlier in the chapter.

Music has been found to alter mood in people with dementia. One study showed greater lucidity and focus after engagement in a singing group, within and between sessions of a 6-week intervention [35]. Relatedly, active engagement with music and listening to music have been found to reduce agitation (e.g. repetitive acts, wandering, restlessness, and aggressive behaviours) and behavioural problems in people with dementia [67]. Depression is one of the most prevalent consequences of dementia in older adults, associated with distress, increased cognitive and functional impairment.

A randomised controlled study explored the impact of music on those living with dementia and depression in aged care [66] under four conditions: group music therapy (GMT), recreational choir singing (RCS), combined GMT and RCS, and a control group who received standard care. The participants had a mean age of 86.5 years and 69% were female, which was consistent with the profile of residents in aged care in Australia. Single intervention groups received 2 × 45 min sessions a week for 3 months and then 1 × 45 min for 3 months, and the combined groups received 2 × 45 min in each of GMT and RCS for 3 months and then once a week for each intervention for the remaining 3 months. Participants all had a Clinical Dementia Rating score between 0.5 and 3 (from very mild to moderate) and were also experiencing mild to severe depressive symptoms. Besides standardised measures of depression, proxy, self-reports of a more qualitative nature were also collected.

Tests were undertaken and measured at baseline, after 3 months, after 6 months, and then at 12-month follow-up, with the results revealing RCS had a meaningful reduction in depression and neuropsychiatric measures compared with the control.

GMT had less conclusive results but indicated that it might be more beneficial in later dementia than in earlier stages. Also, although the combined group received double the number of music sessions, it did not produce clear outcomes. The positive benefits of the RCS condition suggest that behavioural aspects such as the social group dynamic, an emphasis on fun and less focus on the individual (potentially greater cognitive load was induced in the GMT sessions) might have fed into the positive outcome [68].

Reviewing this literature it is evident that artistic engagements for older people are now being skilfully developed and appraised in interventions with registered therapists and with experienced community artists. There are many learnings in the research which informs how practices might be refined and developed. Looking to the future, several key topics remain to be addressed.

7.4 Concluding Thoughts

7.4.1 Why Are Creative Ageing Approaches Important?

Creative arts engagements offer routes to cognitive, physical, social/emotional health, and wellbeing. They can stimulate and protect brain function and delay cognitive decline in older people. In the work explored in this chapter, creative arts engagements have been shown to have the capacity to set new challenges, develop new skills, enrich participants' mental lives, and preserve and augment self-identities and social networks. Given the history of creative arts in cultural practices, it seems that all the creative research discussed also has the potential to generate and sustain the expression of cultural belief, aesthetics, and even spirituality. Crucially, cultures across the world integrate artistic practices into rites, rituals for meaning and understanding, though as we have seen in examples from Iceland and Australia, these are perhaps more integrated and recognised in some cultures than others. Despite their impressive potential, however, we tend to overlook creative arts and their importance. Even if we do not engage in formal activities such as singing in choirs or taking dance classes, through incidental practices such as singing along with music in our heads or moving to the beat of music on the radio, we are engaging in small acts of artistic creativity which have been shown to have beneficial impact [22]. Above all, creative arts have multiple touchpoints all affecting us simultaneously, offering support across diverse domains. As people transition towards and through old age, creative arts engagement can be a powerful and enjoyable tool to ameliorate against the physical and cognitive decline that most experience.

7.4.2 The Challenges of Creative Ageing

Despite the exciting potential of creative arts in the context of ageing, there are challenges associated with their development and implementation. These include addressing accessibility, applying circumstance-appropriate approaches, benchmarking and regulating facilitator skill levels, and gathering nuanced evidence.

For some people Creative Ageing programmes are inaccessible. Five dimensions of accessibility have been identified: (1) approachability; (2) acceptability; (3) availability and accommodation; (4) affordability; (5) appropriateness [69]. It is important to find ways to communicate the attributes and benefits of creative arts programmes in a way that acknowledges the barriers associated with each of these dimensions and gives people from all walks of life (social, cultural, gender, disability) the capacity to assess relevance for them, and should they choose to participate, the means to do so. For example, attaching models such as social prescribing to the aged pension and other aged care support schemes would seem an important step towards equity of availability. Similarly, an ongoing policy of developing and refining suitable programmes to match individual or specific group needs through extensive consultation and co-design with older people themselves is likely to have positive benefits (for example, see approaches and questions raised in [70, 71].

There is a rapidly expanding network of arts practitioners eager to explore Creative Ageing and a variety of facilitation approaches have been developed to engage older people in the arts activities. Categories for these approaches include artist-driven, artwork-centred, and process-driven models. The artist-driven model is an approach where the artists present their work as stimuli to initiate conversations or other forms of exploration for older people. A good example of this might be a visual artist who offers a series of works for display in a care home with the objective of stimulating memories, association and/or aesthetic ambience in ways that bring pleasure and positive benefit to the viewer [72, 73]. A similar result could be achieved by encouraging older people to listen to their preferred music to regulate mood or to reflect on past associations. These 'works' can be made available for informal engagement, or they can be used in structured ways by a facilitator who might ask questions to provoke discussion or offer specific ways in which the materials might be used, for example, building a specific kind of playlist for specific outcomes [22]. A second model is where artists themselves work with a group of older people to generate a specific piece of work or event to be presented in a public forum, for example, an exhibition, a play, or a concert (see examples in [74]). This type of work could include challenging ageist stereotypes by demonstrating active, skilled engagement or the work may be designed to provoke public discussion on topical matters such as climate change action. Process-driven approaches typically have therapeutic or problem-solving aims. Therapeutic arts programmes might be designed to improve cognitive/physical functioning, or simply offer relaxation. Problem-solving solutions include using the social processes of a dance group, a community gardening project, or a knitting circle to overcome social isolation. Facilitators with different skills and experiences might work within some or all of these approach models but it is important that they do so reflexively, regularly contemplating whether the approach they are taking remains the best for the circumstances of their engagement.

There is ongoing debate about relevant skills and training for creative arts facilitators. Creative arts therapists undertake graduate level training, usually at master's level and develop skills in psychotherapy utilising creative modalities, including drama, dance, music, and visual art making within a therapeutic relationship. Their practices can range from group community to individual clinical settings. They become eligible for registration to professional therapy associations that have been formed across the globe (e.g. Australian Music Therapy Association, American Dance Therapy Association, and the Hong Kong Association of Art Therapies). Membership involves adhering to a set of standards and professional practices. For community artists, work can be built through experience, though there are now increasing numbers of master's programmes in socially engaged arts practices, community arts, and community cultural development. Teaching qualifications in school or community college education also provide training in understanding theory and gaining skills in delivering and managing group learning. Further specialist development in specific contexts such as working in dementia care is available and enhances skills. These facilitators work within a multi-disciplinary team including gerontologists, physio- and speech therapists, care support staff and diversional or activity support workers, the latter supporting the arts practitioner. However, it may also be that a person works alone as a sole agent, running activities across a range of contexts. Across all these modalities, it is important to develop context-specific benchmarks that allow realisable expectations of appropriate facilitation skill levels to become established.

The research itself also requires more focus around how the creative arts impact including a body of research evidence that comprehensively explores comparisons between different doses and types of activities in order to ascertain optimal benefits with suitable programmes. The principles and practice of co-design requires more careful methodological work to ensure that work can be built from need and delivered for sustainability, which requires more collaboration between all stakeholders.

With more work ahead, Creative Ageing presents as an exciting concept which has much to offer individuals, their communities and society at large. Contributing to the development of practices and policies that support the aspirations of advocates and practitioners will be critical further steps.

References

1. Bradfield E. Subjective experiences of participatory arts engagement of healthy older people and explorations of creative ageing. Public Health. 2021;198:53–8. https://doi.org/10.1016/j.puhe.2021.06.019.
2. Groot B, de Kock L, Liu Y, Dedding C, Schrijver J, Teunissen T, van Hartingsveldt M, Menderink J, Lengams Y, Lindenberg J, Abma T. The value of active arts engagement on health and well-being of older adults: a nation-wide participatory study. Int J Environ Res Public Health. 2021;18(15):8222. https://doi.org/10.3390/ijerph18158222.
3. Noice T, Noice H, Kramer AF. Participatory arts for older adults: a review of benefits and challenges. Gerontologist. 2014;54(5):741–53. https://doi.org/10.1093/geront/gnt138.
4. Joss T, Daykin N. Arts for health and wellbeing: an evaluation framework. London: Public Health England; 2016.
5. Klimczuk A. Creative aging: drawing on the arts to enhance healthy aging. In: Encyclopedia of geropsychology, vol. 2016. Singapore: Springer; 2016. p. 608–12. https://doi.org/10.1007/978-981-287-082-7_363.

6. Phillipson C. Ageing. New York: Wiley; 2013.
7. Brooke E. Creative ageing and the arts of care: reframing active ageing. Bingley: Emerald Publishing; 2022. https://doi.org/10.1108/9781838674359.
8. Hanna G, Perlstein S. Creativity matters: arts and aging in America. Washington DC: American for the Arts; 2008.
9. Finnish Observatory for Arts and Cultural Education [Internet]. Helsinki: University of the Arts Helsinki; 2017. Available from: http://cerada.uniarts.fi/en/observatory.
10. All-Party Parliamentary Group on Arts, Health and Wellbeing Inquiry. Creative health: The arts for health and wellbeing report July 2017 (2nd ed.). England & Wales; All-Party Parliamentary Group on the Arts; 2017.
11. American for the Arts National Conventions and Arts Policy Roundtables https://www.americansforthearts.org/research. Accessed 6 Nov 2022.
12. Commonwealth of Australia (2023). Revive: a place for every story: a story for every place. Australia Council for the Arts; 2022.
13. Australia Council for the Arts. Connected lives: creative solutions to the mental health crisis. Report on the Arts, Creativity and Mental Wellbeing Policy Development Program. Sydney: Australia Council for the Arts; 2022.
14. Jensen A, Bungay H. Swedish primary healthcare practitioners' perspectives on the impact of arts on prescription for patients and the wider society: a qualitative interview study. BMC Health Serv Res. 2021;21(1):1–0. https://doi.org/10.1186/s12913-021-07258-7.
15. Cohen G. The mature mind: the positive power of the aging brain. New York: Basic Books; 2005.
16. Cohen G, Perlstein S, Chapline J, Kelly J, Firth KM, Simmens S. The impact of professionally conducted cultural programs on the physical health, mental health, and social functioning of older adults. Gerontologist. 2006;46(6):726–34. https://doi.org/10.1093/geront/46.6.726.
17. Clift S. The need for robust critique in arts and health evidence reviews: a cautionary tale of an emperor's new clothes. In: Plenary presentation. Performing creativity, culture, and wellbeing conference, The University of Melbourne, 16–17 Feb 2023.
18. Creech A, Hallam S, Varvarigou M, McQueen H, Gaunt H. Active music making: a route to enhanced subjective wellbeing among older people. Perspect Pub Health. 2013;133(1):36–43. https://doi.org/10.1177/1757913912466950.
19. Creech A, Hallam S, Varvarigou M, McQueen H. Active ageing with music: supporting wellbeing for the third and fourth ages. London: Institute of Education, University of London; 2014.
20. Deci EL, Ryan RM. The "what" and "why" of goal pursuits: human needs and the self-determination of behaviour. Psychol Inq. 2000;11(4):227–68. https://doi.org/10.1207/S15327965PLI1104_01.
21. Lee J, Davidson JW, Krause AE. Older people's motivations for participating in community singing in Australia. Int J Commun Music. 2016;9(2):191–206. https://doi.org/10.1386/ijcm.9.2.191_1.
22. Davidson JW, Garrido S. My life as a playlist. Perth: UWA Publishing; 2014.
23. Lawlor R. Voices of the first day: awakening in the Aboriginal dreamtime. Rochester: Inner Traditions International Ltd.; 1991.
24. Sivertsen N, Harrington A, Hamiduzzaman M. Exploring Aboriginal aged care residents' cultural and spiritual needs in South Australia. BMC Health Serv Res. 2019;19(1):477. https://doi.org/10.1186/s12913-019-4322-8.
25. Taylor K, Guerin P. Health care and indigenous Australians—cultural safety in practice. South Yarra: Palgrave Macmillan; 2010.
26. Viscogliosi C, Asselin H, Basile S, Borwick K, Couturier Y, Drolet MJ, Gagnon D, Obradovic N, Torrie J, Zhou D, Levasseur M. Importance of Indigenous elders' contributions to individual and community wellness: results from a scoping review on social participation and intergenerational solidarity. Can J Public Health. 2020;111(5):667–81. https://doi.org/10.17269/s41997-019-00292-3.

27. van der Steen JT, van Soest-Poortvliet MC, van der Wouden JC, Bruinsma MS, Scholten RJ, Vink AC. Music-based therapeutic interventions for people with dementia. Cochrane Database Syst Rev. 2017;5(5):CD003477. https://doi.org/10.1002/14651858.CD003477.pub3. Update in: Cochrane Database Syst Rev. 2018;7:CD003477.
28. Curtis A, Gibson L, O'Brien M, Roe B. Systematic review of the impact of arts for health activities on health, wellbeing and quality of life of older people living in care homes. Dementia. 2018;17(6):645–69. https://doi.org/10.1177/1471301217740960.
29. Van Steenwinkel I, Dierckx de Casterlé B, Heylighen A. How architectural design affords experiences of freedom in residential care for older people. J Aging Stud. 2017;41:84–92. https://doi.org/10.1016/j.jaging.2017.05.001. Epub 2017 May 19
30. Liddle JL, Parkinson L, Sibbritt DW. Purpose and pleasure in late life: conceptualising older women's participation in art and craft activities. J Aging Stud. 2013;27(4):330–8. https://doi.org/10.1016/j.jaging.2013.08.002.
31. Maidment J, Macfarlane S. Older women and craft: extending educational horizons in considering wellbeing. Soc Work Educ. 2011;30(6):700–11. https://doi.org/10.1080/02615479.2011.586568.
32. Pearce E, Launay J, Dunbar RI. The ice-breaker effect: singing mediates fast social bonding. R Soc Open Sci. 2015;2(10):150221. https://doi.org/10.1098/rsos.150221.
33. Davidson JW. Musical participation: expectations, experiences and outcomes. In: Davidson JW, Deliège I, editors. Music and the mind. Oxford: Oxford University Press; 2011. p. 65–87. https://doi.org/10.1093/acprof:osobl/9780199581566.003.0005.
34. Davidson JW, McNamara B, Rosenwax L, Lange A, Jenkins S, Lewin G. Evaluating the potential of group singing to enhance the well-being of older people. Australas J Ageing. 2014;33(2):99–104. https://doi.org/10.1111/j.1741-6612.2012.00645.x.
35. Davidson JW, Almeida RA. An exploratory study of the impact of group singing activities on lucidity, energy, focus, mood and relaxation for persons with dementia and their caregivers. Psychol Well-Being Theory Res Pract. 2014;4:24–37. https://doi.org/10.1186/s13612-014-0024-5.
36. Greaves CJ, Farbus L. Effects of creative and social activity on the health and well-being of socially isolated older people: outcomes from a multi-method observational study. J R Soc Promot Health. 2006;126:134–42.
37. Cutler D. Tackling loneliness in older age: the role of the arts. London: Baring Foundation; 2012. https://doi.org/10.1177/1466424006064303.
38. Southcott J. And as I go, I love to sing: The Happy Wanderers, music and positive ageing. Int J Commun Music. 2009;2(2-3):143–56. https://doi.org/10.1386/ijcm.2.2-3.143_1.
39. Tymoszuk U, Perkins R, Spiro N, Williamon A, Fancourt D. Longitudinal associations between short-term, repeated, and sustained arts engagement and well-being outcomes in older adults. J Gerontol B Psychol Sci Soc Sci. 2020;75(7):1609–19. https://doi.org/10.1093/geronb/gbz085.
40. Tymoszuk U, Perkins R, Fancourt D, Williamon A. Cross-sectional and longitudinal associations between receptive arts engagement and loneliness among older adults. Soc Psychiatry Psychiatr Epidemiol. 2020;55(7):891–900. https://doi.org/10.1007/s00127-019-01764-0.
41. Todd C, Camic PM, Lockyer B, Thomson LJM, Chatterjee HJ. Museum-based programs for socially isolated older adults: understanding what works. Health Place. 2017;48:47–55. https://doi.org/10.1016/j.healthplace.2017.08.005. Epub 2017 Sep 23.
42. Wood EH, Jepson A, Stadler R. Doing and feeling together in older age: self-worth and belonging through social creative activities. Ageing Soc. 2021;2:1–21. https://doi.org/10.1017/S0144686X21001628.
43. Faulkner R. Icelandic men and me: sagas of singing, self and everyday life. Farnham Surrey: Ashgate; 2013.
44. Amer T, Kalender B, Hasher L, Trehub SE, Wong Y. Do older professional musicians have cognitive advantages? PLoS One. 2013;8(8):e71630. https://doi.org/10.1371/journal.pone.0071630.

45. Moussard A, Bermudez P, Alain C, Tays W, Moreno S. Life-long music practice and executive control in older adults: an event-related potential study. Brain Res. 1642;2016:146–53. https://doi.org/10.1016/j.brainres.2016.03.028.
46. Gooding L, Abner EL, Jicha GA, Kryscio RJ, Schmitt FA. Musical training and late-life cognition. J Alzheimer's Dis Other Dementias. 2014;29:333–43. https://doi.org/10.1177/1533317513517048.
47. Hanna-Pladdy B, Gajewski B. Recent and past musical activity predicts cognitive aging variability: direct comparison with general lifestyle activities. Front Hum Neurosci. 2012;6:198. https://doi.org/10.3389/fnhum.2012.00198.
48. Parbery-Clark A, Strait DL, Anderson S, Hittner E, Kraus N. Musical experience and the aging auditory system: implications for cognitive abilities and hearing speech in noise. PLoS One. 2011;6(5):e18082. https://doi.org/10.1371/journal.pone.0018082.
49. Hanna-Pladdy B, MacKay A. The relation between instrumental musical activity and cognitive aging. Neuropsychology. 2011;25(3):378–86. https://doi.org/10.1037/a0021895.
50. Okely JA, Overy K, Deary IJ. Experience of playing a musical instrument and lifetime change in general cognitive ability: evidence from the lothian birth cohort 1936. Psychol Sci. 2022;33(9):1495–508. https://doi.org/10.1177/09567976221092726.
51. Ferreri L, Moussard A, Bigand E, Tillmann B. Music and the ageing brain. In: Thaut M, Hodges D, editors. The Oxford handbook of music and the brain. Oxford: Oxford Library of Psychology; 2018. https://doi.org/10.1093/oxfordhb/9780198804123.013.25.
52. Bugos JA, Perlstein WM, McCrae CS, Brophy TS, Bedenbaugh PH. Individualized piano instruction enhances executive functioning and working memory in older adults. Aging Ment Health. 2007;11(4):464–71. https://doi.org/10.1080/13607860601086504.
53. Fancourt D, Finn S. What is the evidence on the role of the arts in improving health and wellbeing? A scoping review. Health Evidence Network Synthesis Report 67. World Health Organisation: Copenhagen; 2009.
54. Lazarou I, Parastatidis T, Tsolaki A, Gkioka M, Karakostas A, Douka S, Tsolaki M. International ballroom dancing against neurodegeneration: a randomized controlled trial in Greek community-dwelling elders with mild cognitive impairment. Am J Alzheimers Dis Other Dement. 2017;32(8):489–99. https://doi.org/10.1177/1533317517725813.
55. Zhao J, Li H, Lin R, Wei Y, Yang A. Effects of creative expression therapy for older adults with mild cognitive impairment at risk of Alzheimer's disease: a randomized controlled clinical trial. Clin Interv Aging. 2018;13:1313–20. https://doi.org/10.2147/CIA.S161861.
56. Marquez DX, Wilson R, Aguiñaga S, Vásquez P, Fogg L, Yang Z, Wilbur J, Hughes S, Spanbauer C. Regular Latin dancing and health education may improve cognition of late middle-aged and older latinos. J Aging Phys Act. 2017;25(3):482–9. https://doi.org/10.1123/japa.2016-0049.
57. Noice H, Noice T. An arts intervention for older adults living in subsidized retirement homes. Neuropsychol Dev Cogn B Aging Neuropsychol Cogn. 2009;16(1):56–79. https://doi.org/10.1080/13825580802233400.
58. Alain C, Moussard A, Singer J, Lee Y, Bidelman GM, Moreno S. Music and visual art training modulate brain activity in older adults. Front Neurosci. 2019;13:182. https://doi.org/10.3389/fnins.2019.00182.
59. Fancourt D, Steptoe A, Cadar D. Cultural engagement and cognitive reserve: museum attendance and dementia incidence over a 10-year period. Br J Psychiatry. 2018;213(5):661–3. https://doi.org/10.1192/bjp.2018.129.
60. Fancourt D, Steptoe A. Cultural engagement predicts changes in cognitive function in older adults over a 10 year period: findings from the English Longitudinal Study of Ageing. Sci Rep. 2018;8(1):10226. https://doi.org/10.1038/s41598-018-28591-8.
61. Rehfeld K, Lüders A, Hökelmann A, Lessmann V, Kaufmann J, Brigadski T, Müller P, Müller NG. Dance training is superior to repetitive physical exercise in inducing brain plasticity in the elderly. PLoS One. 2018;13(7):e0196636. https://doi.org/10.1371/journal.pone.0196636.

62. Fusar-Poli L, Bieleninik Ł, Brondino N, Chen XJ, Gold C. The effect of music therapy on cognitive functions in patients with dementia: a systematic review and meta-analysis. Aging Ment Health. 2018;22(9):1097–106. https://doi.org/10.1080/13607863.2017.1348474.
63. Särkämö T, Ripollés P, Vepsäläinen H, Autti T, Silvennoinen HM, Salli E, Laitinen S, Forsblom A, Soinila S, Rodríguez-Fornells A. Structural changes induced by daily music listening in the recovering brain after middle cerebral artery stroke: a voxel-based morphometry study. Front Hum Neurosci. 2014;8:245. https://doi.org/10.3389/fnhum.2014.00245.
64. Dowlen R, Keady J, Milligan C, Swarbrick C, Ponsillo N, Geddes L, et al. The personal benefits of musicking for people living with dementia: a thematic synthesis of the qualitative literature. Arts Health. 2018;10(3):197–212. https://doi.org/10.1080/17533015.2017.1370718.
65. Young R, Camic PM, Tischler V. The impact of community-based arts and health interventions on cognition in people with dementia: a systematic literature review. Aging Ment Health. 2016;20(4):337–51. https://doi.org/10.1080/13607863.2015.1011080.
66. Boersma P, van der Ploeg T, Gobbens RJJ. The added value of art for the well-being of older people with chronic psychiatric illnesses and dementia living in long-term care facilities, and on the collaboration between their caregivers and artists. Healthcare. 2021;9:1489. https://doi.org/10.3390/healthcare9111489.
67. Pedersen SKA, Andersen PN, Lugo RG, Andreassen M, Sütterlin S. Effects of music on agitation in dementia: a meta-analysis. Front Psychol. 2017;8:742. https://doi.org/10.3389/fpsyg.2017.00742.
68. Baker FA, Lee Y-EC, Vieira Sousa T, Stretton-Smith PA, Tamplin J, Sveinsdottir V, Geretsegger M, Dugstad Wake J, Assmus J, Gold C. Clinical effectiveness of music interventions for dementia and depression in elderly care (MIDDEL): Australian cohort of an international pragmatic cluster-randomised controlled trial. Lancet Healthy Longev. 2022;3(3):e153–65. https://doi.org/10.1016/S2666-7568(22)00027-7.
69. Levesque JF, Harris MF, Russell G. Patient-centred access to health care: conceptualising access at the interface of health systems and populations. Int J Equity Health. 2013;12:18. https://doi.org/10.1186/1475-9276-12-18.
70. Goodkind JR, Amer S, Christian C, Hess JM, Bybee D, Isakson BL, Baca B, Ndayisenga M, Greene RN, Shantzek C. Challenges and innovations in a community-based participatory randomized controlled trial. Health Educ Behav. 2017;44(1):123–30. https://doi.org/10.1177/1090198116639243.
71. Gomaa YS, Slade SC, Tamplin J, Wittwer JE, Gray R, Blackberry I, Morris ME. Therapeutic dancing for frail older people in residential aged care: a thematic analysis of barriers and facilitators to implementation. Int J Aging Hum Dev. 2020;90(4):403–22. https://doi.org/10.1177/0091415019854775.
72. Knowles JG, Cole AL, McNiff S. Handbook of the arts in qualitative research: perspectives, methodologies, examples and issues. Thousand Oaks: Sage; 2008. https://doi.org/10.4135/9781452226545.
73. Sullivan G. Artistic thinking as a transcognitive practice: a reconciliation of the process-product dichotomy. Vis Arts Res. 2001;27(2):2–12.
74. Davidson JW, Leske B. Effects of singing on social support and wellbeing among marginalised communities. In: Heydon R, Fancourt D, Cohen A, editors. The Routledge companion to interdisciplinary studies in singing volume III: wellbeing. New York: Routledge; 2020. https://doi.org/10.4324/9781315162546-12.

Memories, Meaning, and Identity

8

Elena Bendien and Tineke Abma

8.1 Introduction

It is March 2022. In the Netherlands, the COVID-19 safety regulations have finally been lifted and Elena (first author) takes the opportunity to call for a meeting with the initiators and volunteers of the free-of-charge reminiscence newspaper in the Southern Dutch province of Zeeland. She wants to know how the women with whom she worked so intensively for 16 months—and who stood at the cradle of the newspaper—are doing, and how the newspaper is received by older people. The newspaper, which is called 'Zeeuws Weerzien', prints materials from archives and reminiscences of people who live or used to live in Zeeland. The aim of this initiative is to bring people together for a lively conversation about their past and present everyday life experiences. The idea for the newspaper came up in 2018, during a project, which was based on participatory action research (PAR) [1, 2] and aimed at active involvement of community-dwelling older adults in reminiscence sessions [3].

Six women volunteers, between 57 and 89 years old, are present at the meeting in March 2022; three of them were co-researchers for the PAR-project in 2018. Elena asks the group to share their thoughts about the value of the reminiscence newspaper for the older population of Zeeland and to think about the factors that contributed to its success (see: Bendien et al. 2022 [3]). The conversation is animated, filled with jokes and joy of seeing each other again. The interaction is lively, but somehow repeatedly 'slips' away from the main topic (the newspaper) to the domain of personal reminiscences. At first Elena tries to stay on track and stick to

E. Bendien (✉)
Leyden Academy on Vitality and Ageing, Leiden, The Netherlands

T. Abma
Leyden Academy on Vitality and Ageing, Leiden University Medical Centre, Leiden, The Netherlands
e-mail: bendien@leydenacademy.nl; abma@leydenacademy.nl

J. Byles (ed.), *What Matters for Healthy Ageing*, Topics in Geriatric Care, https://doi.org/10.1007/978-981-96-0462-3_8

her plan, but eventually she gives in to the spontaneous flow of recollections about recent and past events that the volunteers come up with. Their relationship has always been one of mutual learning and Elena wants to continue in that spirit. She is fascinated by the content of the memories the volunteers share, but even more so by the *process* of remembering and the *reflections* on this process.

Martha (89) shares her concern that reminiscing has become more challenging to her because the people who can understand and endorse her memories are passing away. Rose reflects on a strikingly different view which her sister and herself have about their childhood together. She is sad because, in her opinion, her sister's way of remembering their common past doesn't do justice to the efforts that their parents made to raise them well. Then the conversation changes course again and now spirals around the topic of emotionally charged memories and whether or not people should deal with those on their own. Jane (57) suggests that a painful memory that is shared can be met with a response from the group and then lead to a collective feeling of healing. And so, the conversation continues; the participants forget about the time, going back and forth in time, and using their personal recollections in a collective process of remembering and reflections on that process. The topics follow one another, shedding light on past experiences in which various changes in their identities are reflected: 'I think that I may feel proud of what I have become, if I look at what I used to be', says one of the participants. Their (self-)recognition gives them a feeling of belonging and a new experience of a day worth remembering.

This extract illustrates multiple aspects of the remembering process in later life and its potential for a lively interaction, during which the participants engage in collective inquiry about the content and the relational aspects of the process of remembering. All the participants are curious, not only about their past but also about how they remember it. Herein we can see at least one part of their identity reflected: each of them is eager to learn and grow. They ask intriguing questions and are united in that endeavour. This chapter examines why remembering in later life matters, by addressing two questions: (i) how do personal and collective remembering practices in later life at the same time challenge and empower identity, and (ii) how can remembering contribute to healthy and meaningful ageing? We first introduce the theoretical framework within which, based on philosophical interpretations, memory and identity are understood as processes, followed by a focus on remembering as a social practice, based on an interplay between personal and collective memories. This interplay is illustrated with several examples of empirical research with older adults. In the reflection on these examples, both the advantages and challenges of the remembering process in relation to ageing will be discussed, as well as the vital role of the remembering process to maintain one's identity and to age well.

8.2 A Process Approach to Memory and Identity

We often praise people whose memory allows them to remember large pieces of information in great detail. If an older person demonstrates such a cognitive ability, we believe that their (mental) health is in a good state. Based on that, healthy ageing can be defined based on the scope of memories that one can reproduce and on their factual precision. There is however another possibility to relate healthy ageing to memory. Healthy ageing is rooted in what Machteld Huber and colleagues call positive health, i.e. 'the ability to adapt and self-manage in the face of social, physical and emotional challenges' [4 p. 343]. In other words, knowing that biological ageing entails various forms of decline, we assume that healthy ageing involves the ability to deal with these processes without losing meaning in later life. In relation to memory and ageing well, this definition allows us to shift the emphasis from having a well-functioning memory to the ability of participating in the social practice of remembering. We have shown how this works in the excerpt from the lively conversation about past experiences in the introduction: the participants joined in and enjoyed the collective process of remembering.

The capacity to remember factual information tempts us to compare memory with a large (digital) archive that can be accessed by anybody who possesses the proper cognitive or technical tools. Such a visualisation is based on the notion that memories are unchangeable: once they are saved they will remain set until we call upon them in the present. This image of how we can retrieve memories may be true for specific types of information, like the date of certain events or the number of participants during past events, but the way we remember our experiences can be quite different. Based on the interpretation of the remembering process as presented by the French philosopher Henry Bergson, our memory can better be understood as a constant flux of new experiences that are being added to the existing ones, whereby the totality of our memory changes all the time. More specifically, each new experience changes what we know about the world, and irrespective of how small this change may be, all our experiences and the way we understand and interpret them will change as well [5]. This is a challenging way to interpret memory, since it questions its permanency and in fact, the authenticity of our experiences. Yet, if we accept that our memory is subject to a constant process of change, then it will allow us to understand that experiences which are reconstructed during the remembering process are the experiences of *the person in the present* and not of the person from the past. Rose, from our opening example, remembers her childhood not as the carefree child she used to be, but as an adult woman, equipped by life-long experiences and a moral code that she developed during her life. That is why her recollection is guided by a feeling of respect and gratitude towards her parents, which she finds important to emphasise in face of her sister's memories, that diverge from her own. Indeed, memories are the outcome of a hermeneutic process of meaning making, and perspectives on the past may deviate or conflict.

Understanding memory as a process allows us to interpret identity in terms of a process as well. We do not identify memory with identity, but we can consider human experiences as fruitful soil on which identity can thrive [6]. The loss of these experiences can challenge the coherency of a person's self-story and can lead to a change in identity as well [7]. Recent studies on identity and neurodegenerative diseases address various factors that can influence the identity of an affected person. A phenomenological study demonstrates that a loss of memory does not necessarily lead to a total loss of identity because human bodies can still have memories and maintain the self-awareness of the affected person [8]. The work of medical clowns in dementia care is often based on the same principals, i.e. regarding the body as a site of memory [9]. A study that has taken the 'essential-moral-self' approach, argues that identity is rather rooted in the moral faculty of a person than in his memories, based on a third-person judgement. If this moral faculty changes, as may take place due to the Alzheimer disease, the person seems to become somebody else [10]. Yet another study explores whether a loss of memory due to the Alzheimer disease, semantic dementia, or frontotemporal dementia actually leads to a diminished sense of self [11]. The authors come to conclusion that there is no evidence of a global loss of self, and there are various mechanisms that allow for at least partial restoration of a temporal self-narrative. These studies, quite different in their approaches, confirm the importance of any human experience to the integrity of one's identity. They also suggest that identity can be characterised by a certain degree of plasticity, or even adaptability in the face of disease or other life events.

According to our process approach, identity is related to various capacities and types of memory and undergoes changes during the entire life course. As social scientists we are especially interested in how identity can be actualised through various forms of interaction with others. Identity as we understand it is subject to change in the same way that memory is. Being inspired by Michel Foucault, we approach identity not as a substance but as 'a form, and this form is not primarily or always identical to itself' [12, p. 290]. This form depends on various relationships, may have different reference points in people's lives, and therefore is not singular [13]. Think about Rose again, whom we learn through her recollection as a daughter of her parents, as a sister, and as a grown-up woman who is doing voluntary work, all at the same time. Her identity presents itself in various forms, which feed on various old and new experiences and on her moral code. Understanding identity as changing is a daring approach because our common sense seeks verification of the fact that 'I know who I am', rather than being open to a constant challenge of discovering "who I am becoming'. Yet, as our illustrations of the remembering process will show, a coherent version of ourselves and therefore our wellbeing can benefit more from accepting the changing nature of memory and identity than from the notion of permanency of our experiences and ourselves, especially where wellbeing and meaning in later life are concerned.

8.3 Remembering as a Social Practice

Our process approach towards memory and identity defines our epistemological perspective. We investigate remembering as a social practice. We study memory, identity, and ageing in relation to each other, and we focus on how remembering in later life can bring about a positive change in the lives of older people. Our focus is on everyday remembering in interaction [14]. The perspectives of the older people themselves are central to our approach, which is why our empirical data are derived from participatory research with older people.

Remembering is reconstructive by nature, it is based on our multiple experiences from the past, which we can use as templates or frames that are filled in during the remembering process itself [5, 15]. According to the French philosopher and sociologist Maurice Halbwachs, we never remember as isolated individuals [16]. In its essence remembering can never represent a strictly individual process; it is a social practice, deeply rooted in our relationships and interactions with others. To paraphrase, we do not remember as an isolated individual, we remember in the context of our relational networks with others: as a daughter or a son of the family, as a student at school, as a member of a sport club, etc. Our social roles and the respective 'forms' of our identity, define what and how we remember, and we need others in order to confirm, verify, and complete our recollections. Halbwachs was the first to introduce the notion of collective memory and to describe the interplay between personal and collective memories. Collective memory can be a powerful ideological tool for sense making of important historical events [17], but it is also an important means for a personal feeling of belonging if there remains space for individual interpretation of the collective memory [18]. Collective remembering stimulated by reminiscence interventions can be also an important source of empowerment and contribute to a better health in later life [19].

8.4 Remembering and Ageing

In their book, Nussbaum and Levmore [20] discuss the widespread notion that older people often dwell on the past. They find it not surprising, considering the lifespan of older people: more years lie behind them than ahead. Yet, the authors show convincingly that concentrating solely on the past can lead to escapism, depression, and even self-destructive behaviour. At the same time neglecting the past can have negative consequences for a coherent feeling of one's identity as well. It would seem that having a proper balance between the past, the present, and the future perspectives in one's life is a condition for healthy ageing [21]. Given the social nature of the remembering process, others can help us to reach this balance.

In our work, we acknowledge a difference between remembering as a basic, spontaneous or mediated, human practice which takes place in everyday life, and reminiscence work as an intervention for (older) persons, developed with a specific purpose: to stimulate the memory function of older people and to promote their interaction and wellbeing [22]. We use remembering and reminiscing as interchangeable terms, except for cases where reference is made explicitly to reminiscence work as intervention.

The empirical material we use in this chapter illustrates various remembering practices among older adults. Remembering at a later age is not necessarily different from the way (younger) adults engage with it. Nevertheless, one might speak about specific functions and meanings that remembering has in old age, like acknowledgement of the changes that people have experienced during their life course and acceptance of a new version of self [23]. The eight functions of reminiscence/remembering proposed by Webster in 1997 are still actual today: bitterness revival, boredom reduction, conversation, death preparation, identity, intimacy maintenance, problem solving, teaching/informing [24]. Based on these, older people can engage in remembering because they experience it as a pleasurable activity. It can be instrumental, when they want to share their experiences with somebody from the younger generation or it can be obsessive, when they dwell on a dramatic experience from the past. Each instance of remembering can be related to several functions simultaneously, but whatever functions may lie at the basis of the act of remembering, they will tell us something about the wishes and needs of the person who is engaging with remembering in the present. It also allows us to understand the connection between remembering and ageing well.

We shall use several illustrations in order to support the key issues that were discussed so far, namely, how the remembering process itself becomes more important than the retrieved memories, how a diversity of versions about the past may coexist, based on an interplay between a personal and a collective memory, and what remembering can mean for the self-image of an older adult.

8.5 Context of Research

All illustrations are either derived from the transcript of the dialogue session with the volunteers that has been introduced at the beginning of the chapter or from the PAR research project and its spin-off that was carried out in the Netherlands in 2017–2018 [3]. The spin-off is a still ongoing independent initiative, which the authors are now following from a distance. The PAR-project was carried out with Festival of Recognition, a voluntary organisation that was founded in 2014 to organise reminiscence sessions for older people living in long-term care facilities in Zeeland. The sessions are held with the use of 'travel-bags', which are sets of old-fashioned artefacts that are grouped thematically. For example, there are sets called 'School', 'On the beach', or 'In the shop', where paraphernalia are collected that are related to the topic in question. At first, the reminiscence sessions were held for residents of nursing homes. During the research project, the team of volunteers searched for possibilities to extend the activities, by involving community-dwelling older adults in the sessions as well. And then the idea for a free-of-charge reminiscence newspaper was born. The newspaper uses archive material about the province of Zeeland as well as reminiscences of local residents. The data from the research project includes the reports of the reminiscence sessions that were held by older volunteers for people with dementia living in long-term care facilities and for community-dwelling older people. The data from the spin-off project come from public responses to the free-of-charge reminiscence newspaper that continues to be published periodically to date (Picture 8.1).

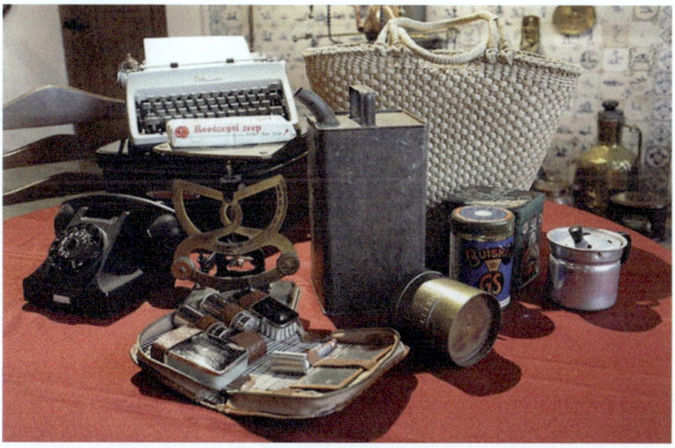

Picture 8.1 Photograph by Karin den Boer, 2018

8.6 The Value of Shared Remembering

Working with older adults in various research settings and projects, we see that collective remembering can be of great importance to older people because their networks inevitably thin out and their losses tend to put pressure on their feeling of belonging. The following story, that was told by one of the volunteers, is characteristic for many visits to a nursing home:

> Volunteer 1: During one of the visits to the nursing home, I met a man. We were just chatting, and he said: "I don't know anyone here'. I asked: 'Where are you from?' He said: 'Limburg'. [another Dutch province] Then he asked me: 'Do you know anything about Limburg?' And then he started singing a song about how beautiful our Limburg is. And he started crying. It stuck with me. I think, people have so many emotions! And this is so difficult for him, precisely because he doesn't feel recognized as a Limburger by the others.

This example provides us with an illustration of what somebody might remember, how remembering takes place, and what it means to this person. The memory itself, mediated by the song about the province where the man comes from, can be called a happy memory. He seems to be proud of Limburg and the song helps him to express that feeling. The challenge that the man is facing is that he finds himself alone with his memories about the past. In his opinion, there is nobody there to share his memories with, and when he reminisces alone, it appears he is experiencing a double loss, the loss of the background he came from and the loss of the possibility to reminisce with others who share similar experiences. In other words, he misses both the feeling of belonging and the process of collective remembering. The volunteer manages to break through his social isolation by asking him about Limburg, so he starts singing about his beloved province.

Another story supports the idea that the process of remembering can be much more important to older people than the remembered item itself:

> Volunteer 2: I was at [place], where we are working with a large group of older residents. We do a lot with them: we work with some old pictures, we read aloud and sometimes we

> sing. Once, during the break, I walked past those people in wheelchairs, asking whether they wanted to hear a special song. And it turned out they all wanted to hear the song about the dead soldier. That is such a sad song, terrible! They all wanted to hear that song. And the next time we were there, they wanted to hear it again! A deeply sad song, about a dead soldier in a church. Well, I'd never heard of it, but I looked it up on YouTube. It's a beautiful song, but your tears would run down your face, truly. But they were all very happy! We had something sweet to go with the coffee and tea. So they were actually having lots of fun. I don't understand why they wanted to hear that sad song.

Comparing this story to the first example, we can understand the confusion of the volunteer. The song that the residents want to hear is sad, but the experience during this collective reminiscence session is described in terms of having fun. By reminiscing together people engage in an activity that unites them as knowers of the past. It gives them authority. During such reminiscence sessions, the saddest memories from the past can be placed into perspective. They recognise the song and feel recognised by others, which gives meaning to their collective experience.

8.6.1 Reflection

Putting these examples in the perspective of healthy ageing allows us to better understand why older people may be willing to engage in reminiscing and which type of reminiscing can bring more satisfaction to their lives. Reminiscences can help to engage with fertile sources of one's identity, like the places where the person used to live, habits they used to have or people they used to know. This is what in the literature is called localisation of experience, i.e. its attachment to a specific territory, place, or even an object [26, 27]. These reminiscences can give a boost to one's life story, but when there is nobody to hear and to share these reminiscences, the exercise may turn into a challenge and result in a feeling of loss. At the same time, the process of collective remembering, can reinforce the feeling of belonging, irrespective of the kind of memories people are sharing [28]. In both cases, we see that remembering is a way of expressing one's identity, which can be experienced as a lonely process or turn into a collective enjoyment.

8.7 'Authenticity' of Memories and Remembering

A challenge to reminisce in later life can occur not only because there are less people around with whom one can share similar memories, but also because the stories which different people remember do not always line up. Collective remembering does not always go as smoothly as in the example with the song about the dead soldier. We saw this in the introductory example, where Rose and her sister turn out to have completely different memories about their childhood. Rose has good memories about her early years, whereas her sister remembers her childhood as an unhappy time. Rose finds that disturbing. Other volunteers confirm that Rose's example is not an exception:

> Volunteer 3: My brother blames me for not noticing all the bad things he saw. He says I should have [seen them] because I was three years older. My brother is a boy, I am a girl. That already gives a different perspective. He experienced things very differently. It's interesting to talk about it.

One of the other volunteers adds that she grew up in a family with 12 siblings, each of whom remembers their childhood differently. The question is whether or how these differences can be of importance to people who share their memories. The reminiscence newspaper could have some answers to this question. The newspaper was designed as a low-hierarchy platform where the authenticity of the reminiscences is concerned. Immediately after the first issue, there was a steady stream of reactions to the published material from the readers; most of them were older inhabitants of Zeeland. Many of them praise this initiative. Others react to a topic that was addressed in a publication, providing additional information or a different view on the matter. The following example is indicative for the discussion about 'true' memories and their meaning to people who share them. In the eighth edition of the newspaper, published in December 2020, there was an article about a dentist practice in the city of Goes, in Zeeland (see Picture 8.2).

The dentist is described as a good specialist and an active citizen, by a former patient who visited him as a child. At the same time, this former patient describes his fear for the treatment, which he attributes to the dentist's lack of patience and general child-unfriendly approach. The article reflects the author's uneasiness, and

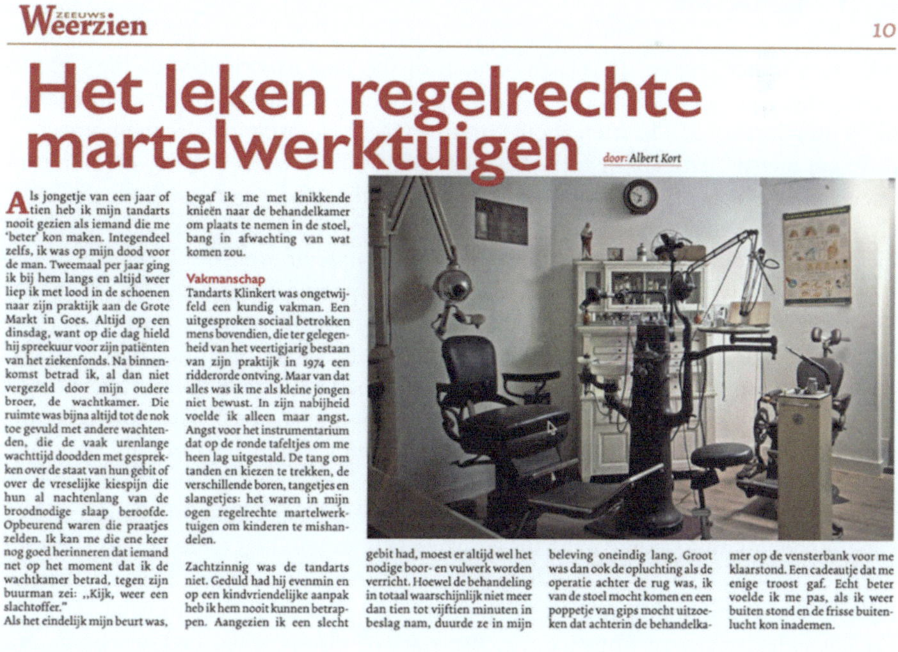

Zeeuws Weerzien 10

Het leken regelrechte martelwerktuigen

door: Albert Kort

Als jongetje van een jaar of tien heb ik mijn tandarts nooit gezien als iemand die me 'beter' kon maken. Integendeel zelfs, ik was op mijn dood voor de man. Tweemaal per jaar ging ik bij hem langs en altijd weer liep ik met lood in de schoenen naar zijn praktijk aan de Grote Markt in Goes. Altijd op een dinsdag, want op die dag hield hij spreekuur voor zijn patiënten van het ziekenfonds. Na binnenkomst betrad ik, al dan niet vergezeld door mijn oudere broer, de wachtkamer. Die ruimte was bijna altijd tot de nok toe gevuld met andere wachtenden, die de vaak urenlange wachttijd doodden met gesprekken over de staat van hun gebit of over de vreselijke kiespijn die hun al nachtenlang van de broodnodige slaap beroofde. Opbeurend waren die praatjes zelden. Ik kan me die ene keer nog goed herinneren dat iemand net op het moment dat ik de wachtkamer betrad, tegen zijn buurman zei: ,,Kijk, weer een slachtoffer."
Als het eindelijk mijn beurt was, begaf ik me met knikkende knieën naar de behandelkamer om plaats te nemen in de stoel, bang in afwachting van wat komen zou.

Vakmanschap

Tandarts Klinkert was ongetwijfeld een kundig vakman. Een uitgesproken sociaal betrokken mens bovendien, die ter gelegenheid van het veertigjarig bestaan van zijn praktijk in 1974 een ridderorde ontving. Maar van dat alles was ik me als kleine jongen niet bewust. In zijn nabijheid voelde ik alleen maar angst. Angst voor het instrumentarium dat op de ronde tafeltjes om me heen lag uitgestald. De tang om tanden en kiezen te trekken, de verschillende boren, tangetjes en slangetjes: het waren in mijn ogen regelrechte martelwerktuigen om kinderen te mishandelen.

Zachtzinnig was de tandarts niet. Geduld had hij evenmin en op een kindvriendelijke aanpak heb ik hem nooit kunnen betrappen. Aangezien ik een slecht gebit had, moest er altijd wel het nodige boor- en vulwerk worden verricht. Hoewel de behandeling in totaal waarschijnlijk niet meer dan tien tot vijftien minuten in beslag nam, duurde ze in mijn beleving oneindig lang. Groot was dan ook de opluchting als de operatie achter de rug was, ik van de stoel mocht komen en een poppetje van gips mocht uitzoeken dat achterin de behandelkamer op de vensterbank voor me klaarstond. Een cadeautje dat me enige troost gaf. Echt beter voelde ik me pas, als ik weer buiten stond en de frisse buitenlucht kon inademen.

Picture 8.2 The article in the newspaper Zeeuws Weerzien, edition December 2020. Title: They seemed like real torture devices the storyteller describes himself as a 'victim'. The newspaper received two reactions to the article:

> Reader 1: That gentleman [the author of the article] must have had a bad time during his younger years. I had that dentist for years, with four small children. And I never noticed that he was impatient or annoying. I found him really child-friendly. My children weren't afraid of him either, so you can see that every person reacts differently.
>
> Reader 2: When people suffered from toothache [gives the name of tooth pain in a dialect of Zeeland], they did not go to the dentist but to the doctor because the dentist was a non-existent figure in most villages. The doctor asked to show the painful spot.
>
> You pointed with your finger where the tormentor was situated. The doctor grabbed a pair of forceps and pulled the tooth out of your mouth, without anaesthesia of course.

In the first reaction, the published information is refuted, in the second it is put into perspective. Together the three recollections can be called collective remembering. In this case, providing your own version of the past can feel very important to the reader. We can argue that the meaning of this exchange is not only to distinguish right from wrong, but also to share your own experience with others. So, the reminiscence newspaper is creating a platform, where a variety of versions of the past can be articulated and coexist. As Jane, the initiator of the newspaper, put it: 'We invite people to tell their own stories about Zeeland. And this makes each story OK in advance'.

8.7.1 Reflection

'OK in advance' means that each version of the past experience has the right to exist, where personal memories are concerned. The debate about 'true' memories has a long history and is often about controversies as a result of false memories or a different interpretation of historical events [29]. Dealing with everyday memories in later age, we accept that there is a diversity within the accounts about the past. Hence, we use diversity as an explanatory framework in order to understand the differences in our recollections about the same people or events.

We accept without questioning the fact that people have different identities. Therefore, it should be no surprise that they may remember things differently. The issue connecting the authenticity of memories with ageing well lies in the acceptance by other people of your own version of the past [30]. In fact, it is important to one's wellbeing to be able to have your own version of the past. This is what reminiscence sessions can bring about, namely different stories, inspired by the same old-fashioned artefacts. The reminiscence newspaper facilitates the same process but more explicitly: it highlights a newspaper article from the archive or a personal experience, inviting people in an unobtrusive way to tell their (side of the) story. In terms of healthy ageing, the newspaper opens a possibility for an inclusive interaction, where each opinion counts. The newspaper gives an answer to what Miranda Fricker calls epistemic injustice, i.e. the state of affairs when certain people are deprived of the right to be carriers of knowledge. Their voices cannot be heard and therefore their experiences remain unknown to others [31]. The reminiscence newspaper treats everybody as a knower and therefore restores epistemic justice, which is one of the main factors of its success.

8.8 Selves We Remember

By means of spontaneous or mediated remembering, older people can reconstruct not only various experiences from the past, but earlier forms of their own selves as well. Our data shows that becoming older can influence one's self-perception and the manner in which people engage with their reminiscences. Martha, the oldest of the volunteers, explained:

> Reminiscing felt different when I was 80. When you become 85 or 90, something changes in the way you think. There are less people around from the same age group. I think you must approach these people in a different way. They often stay at home. I myself prefer to meet people who are younger. But I don't know for how long they will want to meet me.

The last remark demonstrates how internalised ageism can undermine the self-confidence of this older person and to which extent it can influence her health and wellbeing [32]. The reference to changes in one's personality that people experience when they become older, is not just an illustration of the theoretical point that has been made above, namely that our identity is better understood in terms of plurality of forms, than as an unchangeable entity. Acknowledgment of the changes in one's identity can be a key to accepting ageing and the changes that it brings about as well [23]. The volunteers working with the reminiscence newspaper explain how ageing and changes in one's identity juxtapose during everyday remembering practices, which they observe or experience themselves:

> Volunteer 2: When I remember myself as a child, then I think: it [change] does not matter, does it? If you are sober enough and honest enough with yourself, you should be able to see that you have changed after all. This is how I've developed, this is my personality.

The participants of the dialogue session, when asked explicitly what they think about their identity when they remember the past, explain that when they remember a younger self, this can evoke melancholic or even painful memories. At the same time, they nourish the life path they have covered so far and all the changes they lived through, becoming the person they are in the present. One of the topics related to healthy ageing that they address is self-care. Not self-care in the sense of physical vitality, but self-care at a more profound level, i.e. care for your younger self:

> Volunteer 3: If I could I'd send that kid that I used to be, a note: 'Oh, don't worry too much. It's really going to be okay'.

Once again, different forms of the self are made explicit during the remembering process. Moreover, the volunteer looks through a lens of wisdom and care at her younger self, almost like a mother who is trying to protect this child against disappointments and worries of the life that lies ahead.

8.8.1 Reflection

The assumptions regarding the unchangeability of memory and identity can become a source of mental and even physical distress in later life. Understanding memories as unchangeable leaves no space for renegotiation of our past experiences and no flexibility to accept the changes that people undergo [33]. That is why our conceptualisation of memory and identity is based on a process approach and that is why we see the potential for continuing development and growth, but also reconciliation, irrespective of one's chronological age [23].

The last examples show how acceptance of changes can become an important means in addressing ageism and self-ageism. When left unaddressed, self-ageism can have negative consequences on the mental and physical health and wellbeing of older adults [34, 35]. Reminiscing, not only with your peers but also with younger people, can have a positive influence on ageing well for both parties [36].

The positive aspect of knowledge transfer is often raised when remembering takes place in mixed groups. Other examples of intergenerational interaction can be seen when each party has something to share and something to learn [37]. Involvement with new people, new skills and new insights can tempt older adults to look forward and make plans for the future.

Acceptance of the changes that one has gone through in one's personal development, can be seen as a first step on the way towards anti-ageism and can help to address self-ageism [25]. If an older person can look back with love and care to the younger self, as the last example points out, then it allows you to love—or at least to accept—your older self as well. Remembering practices in old age can form an integral part of ageing well, when they are seen not as a time machine to revive the past, but as a lively means for interaction in the present and for planning the future (Picture 8.3).

8.9 Concluding Notes

In this chapter, we explored how memory, meaning, and identity are interconnected in old age, and how remembering in later life is a personal and collective process of meaning making, which can empower and contribute to healthy and meaningful ageing. We used examples from a participatory research project and a dialogue session among volunteers in reminiscence practices to illustrate the power of collective remembering in old age. A key finding we brought to the fore is the value of *shared* remembering. If people share their memories jointly, then this can strengthen their feeling of belonging and generate joy, irrespective of the kind of memories they are sharing. If on the other hand, there is no one to listen, the reminiscences may turn into a challenge and result in a feeling of loss.

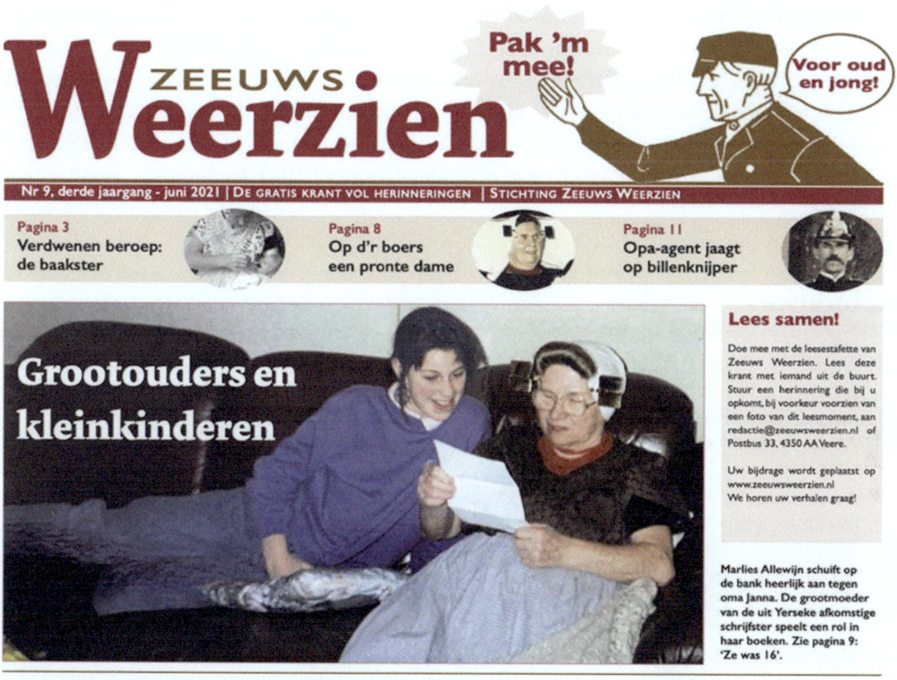
Zeeuws Weerzien

Pak 'm mee!

Voor oud en jong!

Nr 9, derde jaargang - juni 2021 | De gratis krant vol herinneringen | Stichting Zeeuws Weerzien

Pagina 3
Verdwenen beroep: de baakster

Pagina 8
Op d'r boers een pronte dame

Pagina 11
Opa-agent jaagt op billenknijper

Grootouders en kleinkinderen

Lees samen!

Doe mee met de leesestafette van Zeeuws Weerzien. Lees deze krant met iemand uit de buurt. Stuur een herinnering die bij u opkomt, bij voorkeur voorzien van een foto van dit leesmoment, aan redactie@zeeuwsweerzien.nl of Postbus 33, 4350 AA Veere.

Uw bijdrage wordt geplaatst op www.zeeuwsweerzien.nl
We horen uw verhalen graag!

Marlies Allewijn schuift op de bank heerlijk aan tegen oma Janna. De grootmoeder van de uit Yerseke afkomstige schrijfster speelt een rol in haar boeken. Zie pagina 9: 'Ze was 16'.

Picture 8.3 Zeeuws Weerzien, edition 9, June 2021

A second key finding is that the 'authenticity' of memories and its link with healthy ageing lies in the acceptance that everyone has their own version of the past. Even stronger, it is important to one's wellbeing to be able to have your own version of the past. This is what reminiscence sessions can bring about, namely different stories inspired by the same old-fashioned artefacts. This way of working contributes to what Miranda Fricker [30] calls 'epistemic justice.' Each and every person should have the possibility to witness and interpret his or her past and not be excluded from the process of remembering and knowledge production.

The third key finding is that remembering can contribute to the development and growth of one's identity, irrespective of one's chronological age. If an older person can care about the younger self, then it should enable that person to accept the older self as well, which we see as an important step towards self-age friendliness.

The examples above also demonstrate that the fun-parts of remembering in later life coexist with the challenges, when people feel alone, feel a loss, or simply feel old. Many of the volunteers find that older people have a certain knowledge that can be shared with others, and that their skills should not be wasted, just because they have reached a certain chronological age. This reflection brings us to the important notion of what can be understood by ageing well.

All older people with whom we have worked in our projects experienced physical signs of ageing. When observing the everyday remembering practices and also the organised reminiscence sessions, we find that remembering, whether it is linked to happy or to sad memories, shared with others or questioned by them, articulated with words or transmitted emotionally, forms an intrinsic part of what can be called ageing well. In fact, this process is so important, that we consider it to be a human right. It is not the number of memories that one can recall or their exactness, that matter most for the process of remembering as a human practice. Remembering creates the possibility to experience healthy ageing and to have a meaningful later life.

References

1. Abma TA, Cook T, Rämgård M, Kleba E, Harris J, Wallerstein N. Social impact of participatory health research: collaborative non-linear processes of knowledge mobilization. Educ Action Res. 2017;25(4):489–505. https://doi.org/10.1080/09650792.2017.1329092.
2. Abma T, Banks S, Cook T, Dias S, Madsen W, Springett J, Wright MT. Participatory research for health and social well-being. Cham: Springer; 2019.
3. Bendien E, Groot B, Abma T. Circles of impacts within and beyond participatory action research with older people. Ageing Soc. 2022;42(5):1014–34. https://doi.org/10.1017/S0144686X20001336.
4. Huber M, Knottnerus JA, Green L, Horst HVD, Jadad AR, Kromhout D, Leonard B, Lorig K, Loureiro MI, Meer JWMVD, Schnabel P, Smith R, Weel CV, Smid H. How should we define health? BMJ. 2011;343(2):d4163.
5. Middleton D, Brown SD. The social psychology of experience: studies in remembering and forgetting. London: Sage; 2005.
6. Barclay K, Koefoed NJ. Family, memory, and identity: an introduction. J Fam Hist. 2021;46(1):3–12. https://doi.org/10.1177/0363199020967297.
7. Caddell LS, Clare L. The impact of dementia on self and identity: a systematic review. Clin Psychol Rev. 2010;30(1):113–26. https://doi.org/10.1016/j.cpr.2009.10.00.
8. Fuchs T. Embodiment and personal identity in dementia. Med Health Care Philos. 2020;23(4):665–76. https://doi.org/10.1007/s11019-020-09973-0.
9. Novy C, Thomas R, Garcia L, Gifford W, Grassau P. Using the performance arts to address a "methods gap" in dementia research. Arts Health. 2022:1–14. https://doi.org/10.1080/17533015.2021.1942093.
10. Strohminger N, Nichols S. Neurodegeneration and identity. Psychol Sci. 2015;26(9):1469–79. https://doi.org/10.1177/0956797615592381.
11. Strikwerda-Brown C, Grilli MD, Andrews-Hanna J, Irish M. "All is not lost"—rethinking the nature of memory and the self in dementia. Ageing Res Rev. 2019;54:100932. https://doi.org/10.1016/j.arr.2019.100932.
12. Foucault M. The ethics of the concern for self as a practice of freedom. In: Ethics: essential works of foucault 1954–1984, vol. 1. London: Penguin Books; 2000.
13. Brown SD, Reavey P. Psychology without foundations: history, philosophy and psychosocial theory. London: Sage; 2009.
14. Edwards D, Middleton D. Joint remembering: constructing an account of shared experience through conversational discourse. Discourse Process. 1986;9(4):423–59. https://doi.org/10.1080/01638538609544651.
15. Schwartz B. Abraham Lincoln and the forge of national memory. Chicago: University of Chicago Press; 2003.
16. Halbwachs M. The collective memory. 1st ed. New York: Harper & Row; 1980.
17. Wertsch JV. Voices of collective remembering. Cambridge: Cambridge University Press; 2002.
18. Bendien E. Remembering (in) the past perfect: ethical shifts in times. Memory Stud. 2012;5(4):445–61. https://doi.org/10.1177/1750698012439198.

19. Shropshire M. Reminiscence intervention for community-dwelling older adults without dementia: a literature review. Br J Commun Nurs. 2019;25(1):40–4. https://doi.org/10.12968/bjcn.2020.25.1.40.
20. Nussbaum M, Levmore S. Aging thoughtfully. 1st ed. Oxford: Oxford University Press; 2017.
21. Ferraro KF, Wilkinson LR. Alternative measures of self-rated health for predicting mortality among older people: is past or future orientation more important? Gerontologist. 2015;55(5):836–44. https://doi.org/10.1093/geront/gnt098.
22. Demiray B, Mischler M, Martin M. Reminiscence in everyday conversations: a naturalistic observation study of older adults. J Gerontol B. 2019;74(5):745–55. https://doi.org/10.1093/geronb/gbx141.
23. Bendien [ECA1] EM. From the art of remembering to the craft of ageing (Doctoral dissertation, Amsterdam: Stichting Humanitas). 2010.
24. Webster JD. The reminiscence functions scale: a replication. Int J Aging Hum Dev. 1997;44(2): 137–48. https://doi.org/10.2190/AD4D-813D-F5XN-W07G.
25. Casey ES. Remembering: a phenomenological study. Indiana: Indiana University Press; 1987.
26. Radley A. Artefacts, memory and a sense of the past. In: Middleton D, Edwards D, editors. Collective remembering. London: Sage; 1990;46–59.
27. Pasupathi M, Wainryb C. Remembering good and bad times together: functions of collaborative remembering. In: Meade ML, Harris CB, Bergen PV, Sutton J, Barnier AJ, editors. Collaborative remembering: theories, research, applications. Oxford: Oxford University Press; 2018;261–79.
28. Campbell S. Relational remembering: rethinking the memory wars. Lanham: Rowman & Littlefield; 2003.
29. Henkel LA, Kris A. Collaborative remembering and reminiscence in older adults. In: Meade ML, Harris CB, Bergen PV, Sutton J, Barnier AJ, editors. Collaborative remembering: theories, research, and applications. Oxford: Oxford University Press; 2018;135–56.
30. Fricker M. Epistemic injustice: power and the ethics of knowing. Oxford: Oxford University Press; 2007.
31. Levy B. Breaking the age code. New York: Random House; 2022.
32. Brown SD, Reavey P. Vital memory and affect: living with a difficult past. London: Routledge; 2015.
33. Allen JO, Solway E, Kirch M, Singer D, Kullgren JT, Moïse V, Malani PN. Experiences of everyday ageism and the health of older US adults. JAMA Netw Open. 2022;5(6):–e2217240. https://doi.org/10.1001/jamanetworkopen.2022.17240.
34. Chang ES, Kannoth S, Levy S, Wang SY, Lee JE, Levy BR. Global reach of ageism on older persons' health: a systematic review. PLoS One. 2020;15(1):e0220857. https://doi.org/10.1371/journal.pone.0220857.
35. Gaggioli A, Morganti L, Bonfiglio S, Scaratti C, Cipresso P, Serino S, Riva G. Intergenerational group reminiscence: a potentially effective intervention to enhance elderly psychosocial well-being and to improve children's perception of aging. Educ Gerontol. 2014;40(7):486–98. https://doi.org/10.1080/03601277.2013.844042.
36. Chonody J, Wang D. Connecting older adults to the community through multimedia: an inter-generational reminiscence program. Active Adapt Aging. 2013;37(1):79–93. https://doi.org/10.1080/01924788.2012.760140.
37. Schuurman B, Lindenberg J, Huijg JM, Achterberg WP, Slaets JP. Expressions of self-ageism in four European countries: a comparative analysis of predictors across cultural contexts. Ageing Soc. 2022;42(7):1589–606. https://doi.org/10.1017/S0144686X20001622.

9 Adapting to Change in the Caring Context

Kirsten Moore and Linda Garcia

9.1 Introduction

For older people requiring long-term support due to chronic health conditions, the bulk of care is provided by family members and friends. In 2015, it was estimated that care provided by informal carers to people living with dementia was equivalent to 40 million full-time workers and expected to increase to 65 million by 2030 [1]. Although commonly referred to as 'caregivers', 'carers', 'care partners' or 'informal carers/caregivers', many people who provide this support do not identify as such or may not see their role as outside the realm of being in a supportive relationship or family network. Furthermore, it is important to remember that providing support to their loved ones is only one of the roles in their lives. For the purposes of this chapter, we will use the term carers.

The context of caring is diverse, yet cultural expectations, gender roles and health and care systems influence who is more likely to become a carer. In lower income countries, there are fewer formal social care services and the responsibility of care is more heavily reliant on family members. Cultural expectations can mean that using residential aged care or paid carers is unacceptable and should be provided by the family. The extent to which care is provided by a sole primary carer or a shared network of extended family also varies and may be influenced by culture. Other characteristics of carers such as sex and gender identity, religion, rurality,

K. Moore (✉)
National Ageing Research Institute, The University of Melbourne, Parkville, Melbourne, VIC, Australia

Medicine—Royal Melbourne Hospital, The University of Melbourne, Parkville, Melbourne, VIC, Australia

L. Garcia
School of Health Sciences at the University of Ottawa, Ottawa, ON, Canada
e-mail: linda.garcia@uottawa.ca

J. Byles (ed.), *What Matters for Healthy Ageing*, Topics in Geriatric Care,
https://doi.org/10.1007/978-981-96-0462-3_9

socio-economic status and quality and type of relationship to the person being supported will impact the caring experience. Health and severity of disease of the carer and the person they support will have an important impact. In short, the experiences of caring are as diverse as human experience.

This chapter explores the role of caring and how that may change over time. We highlight key transitions and factors that can impact on the experience of caring and how caring shapes identity. We begin by exploring how people become carers followed by an overview of the health consequences that have been extensively examined in carer research. We follow this by offering an alternative view and exploring the opportunities for growth and flourishing that caring can offer. We look at some of the challenges of accepting and receiving support services including the transition to long-term residential care. The latter part of the chapter explores palliative and end-of-life care before considering life after being a carer.

9.2 Becoming a Carer

Becoming a carer is not always perceived as a natural evolution of one's roles. Some may feel it is a typical part of being in a relationship as either a spouse, parent or child. However, for some it may not feel like a choice but a role that has been imposed on them. There may be no one else available or someone who is already providing care for family members may become the logical choice to take on the care of other family members. The need for care may be sudden, for example, after a severe stroke or fall where someone may require imminent assistance, whereas others may require a more gradual need for additional support, such as when someone has a more slowly progressing chronic health condition. In some cases, living arrangements must be altered such as when a child decides to move in with an ageing parent to provide support.

Spouses/partners and adult children are the most likely to support older adults, with the responsibility more commonly falling to female rather than male offspring [2]. This reflects societal norms and gendered expectations that caring is provided by women—an extension of the childbearing and child-rearing contribution to society. Comparison of male and female carers highlight gendered differences where females provide more hours of care and more personal care [3]. Many carers are also older themselves. For example, in Australia, 51% of carers who are supporting relatives with dementia are over the age of 65 [4].

The extent to which a carer feels that they had a choice in becoming a carer can impact their experiences and satisfaction in the role. When care is not a choice, the role is more likely to be seen as an interruption to life that impacts on the person's identity and quality of life. Becoming a carer can also be seen as a developmental process. Over time the carer may learn more about the health and care system, and this can enable them to access supports that meet their needs.

9.3 The Impact of Caring

Caring for an older adult who is a parent, a spouse or a friend can be overwhelming. We have known for decades that caring for older adults offers challenges to unpaid family members and friends that can lead to physical and mental health problems requiring assistance from our health, technological and social communities. It can impact physical and mental health, employment and work performance as well as relationships. Much attention has been paid to the higher levels of depression and burden amongst carers [5]. Grief and loss amongst carers can also be high but has received less focus in research and support services [6].

Further complicating our understanding of the degree to which the experience will be demanding are factors such as the type of care that is needed, the amount of time required, the pre-existing relationship with the care receiver or the accessibility to resources. Rightfully so, many policies in high-income countries have focussed on reducing the burden that care can have on carers in the hope that carers will not themselves develop health-related problems and be able to continue in their roles as carers. Many psychosocial interventions have been developed including individual and group-based education and counselling interventions showing benefits in reducing depression [7]. Respite care, which aims to give carers a break, is a key approach to supporting carers. Additional benefits occur when interventions are adapted to be culturally responsive [8].

As with so many other issues, the COVID-19 pandemic has had a monumental impact on how we manage our relationships and how we care for others; especially older adults who live with multiple chronic health conditions [9]. The stress of the pandemic has stretched our capacity to deal with many of the pre-existing challenges facing our older populations and those who are involved in their care as unpaid carers. Faced with the added burden of COVID-19, family and friends were tested as they sought to provide support despite reduced, withdrawn or cancelled community respite services and home care. The data on the long-term impact of the pandemic on carers remains to be collected, but we can imagine it will be great [10].

9.4 An Opportunity for Growth and Development

While there has been much research on burden and depression in caring, there has been little attention paid to how and why some carers thrive when faced with these challenges and burdens. The experience of caring is one many will face at some point in their lives. More than ever before, as unveiled by the pandemic, it is time to transform our perceptions of the experiences of caring into a more balanced view that includes strategies to allow carers not just to survive but to thrive under such adverse conditions.

In a US survey of carers, Skufca [11] found that only 16% of respondents were very prepared for their carer role. Yet, despite this and the fact that caring is stressful, 91% of respondents associated positive emotions with being able to help.

Over half of the respondents were also surprised that they felt 'unexpected joy in caregiving'. These findings highlight that we cannot assume that burden or stress will occur for all carers and that burden will not be accompanied by positive experiences of caring.

A report by the Associated Press-National Opinion Research Center [12] revealed that often carers do not worry about their own needs. Most find caring rewarding despite struggling to take care of their own health, using vacation time to care for older adults and dipping into personal finances to address care receiver needs. Kaschowitz and Brandt [13] found differences in caring across different European countries with some experiencing positive impacts on their health and others not. There is some indication that the positive impacts of providing care are mitigated by elements of self-efficacy and personality (e.g. [14–16] the amount of care needed [17] or the types of tasks required [18]). Long durations of caring, common when caring for someone with dementia, can bring simultaneously positive and negative emotions and reactions as families pass through transitions [19]. Rather than focus interventions almost exclusively on the reduction of burden, positive aspects need to be brought to the forefront to help rebalance the discourse on caring and recommend changes to support those who need help to thrive. Learning new skills, becoming an expert carer, establishing a new identity as a carer, reciprocating care, fulfilling cultural norms and expectations, bringing families together and becoming closer to the care recipient are all potential benefits of caring.

There are many possible strategies for easing the demand and impact on carers. One approach is to focus on the care needs of the recipient and provide programmes that help the family carer with care tasks. Another approach is to shift the focus on how carers adapt and the strategies they use. Identifying what brings carers happiness and wellbeing will help them thrive through moments of intense demand such as the COVID-19 pandemic. Since not all carers need help, rather than focus solely on the high-need and high-cost patients as recommended by Shulz et al. [10], we believe there is value in equally focussing on those who do not need help; on understanding their resilience and even their ability to flourish.

9.5 Accessing Support

Enabling carers to flourish requires targeted and individualised supports that are responsive to the needs of the care recipient and carer. Yet availability of programmes for carers of older people varies considerably in different health and aged care systems. Many aged and social care systems have evolved over many years with new initiatives being added as our understanding of the needs of carers grows. While this increases service options, it can also increase the complexity of the service system. Many carers in high-income countries struggle to navigate an increasingly fragmented service system that can contribute to, rather than alleviate burden and stress. As the global population ages, the need for these services increases and governments and programmes may struggle to meet growing demands. In low- and middle-income countries where population ageing is occurring more rapidly, the resources and infrastructure may be insufficient to quickly develop comprehensive supports for older people and their carers.

Accessing services may also be hampered by healthcare professionals and service providers failing to acknowledge the role and information that carers can contribute. Services rightfully should strive to provide individualised and person-centred care, valuing the input and autonomy of the older person. However, in the context of a cognitive impairment and dementia, the carer may provide valuable insights into the care needs of the older adult that the older adult may lack. Often, however, the carer's views and experiences may not be considered in the assessment and diagnosis process.

Depending on how services perceive, the role of carers also influences the type of support available. Twigg and Atkin [20] argue that services often focus on the needs of the care recipient and tend to treat family carers as either resources, co-workers, co-clients or superseded (replaced by services). As a resource or co-worker, carers are viewed as freely available due to family obligations and the definition of a carer is broad to include anyone who can assist the person requiring care. The cared for person is the central focus and services aim to avoid substituting informal care. When carers are viewed as co-clients, they are viewed as clients in their own right. The definition of carer, therefore, becomes very narrow, focusing only on the needs of those heavily burdened by a caring role. This perspective recognises that sometimes meeting the needs of the carer, as in the form of institutional respite, may be at odds with the cared for person's needs. Carers become 'superseded' when there is a conflict of needs between the carer and the cared for and services aim to fully replace the primary carer. Services provided by mainstream agencies tend to focus on the needs of the person with a disability, while services targeting the needs of carers tend to be provided through the voluntary sector.

Respite care is a key component of carer support and can be provided in a variety of formats and settings. It can be provided in a residential setting where the older person stays overnight or for multiple nights or weeks. Day centres can promote social interaction for the older person and a break for the carer. Other respite may include staff coming into the home to support the older person. However, often respite services are not taken up fully and there is a lack of evidence of their overall benefit [21]. The findings to date suggest that while carers appreciate the break, it is important that the older person receives high quality care as well as some benefit. Day centres can provide a meaningful opportunity for social interaction, but some older people may not feel they need support or reject the implication of dependency. Other barriers can include lack of flexibility, cost, inexperienced staff, lack of continuity of staff and bureaucratic processes to access respite care [22].

Emotional and practical support from family and friends can be crucial for supporting carers and supporting their wellbeing. However, carers may be reluctant to ask for help or be considered a burden to others. Peer support through carer support groups provides an informal peer support outside the family and may be more acceptable. The benefits of these groups include offering an avenue for carers to share their experiences, learn from other carers and feel validated by shared experiences. Carer support groups are effective in reducing carer depression and burden and improving social outcomes [23]. However, they may not suit all carers as some may find hearing other people's stories distressing, leading to an increased emotional load. Also, hearing stories of more advanced disease or end of life may raise new fears for carers about what the future may hold. Individual therapies and counselling may be more suitable for some.

9.6 Transition to Long-Term Residential Care

The use and availability of residential aged care, also referred to as nursing home, care home and long-term care, tends to be higher in high-income countries. The need for residential care may indicate a lack of adequate home-based supports. Family carers may find it particularly difficult to maintain care at home for someone with advanced dementia who may have significant care needs. Factors that can increase the need for residential aged care include older age, living alone, having functional and cognitive limitations, hospitalisation and having a lower income [24].

For some family carers, the transition can be a traumatic and stressful one leading to feelings of grief, loss and guilt [25]. Some spouse carers may see it as signifying the end of their marriage as they no longer reside together. Where care needs are high, carers may be encouraged or sometimes feel pressured by healthcare professionals and other family members to place the care recipient in a facility. Conversely, they may also have family and cultural expectations to continue providing care at home at a time when they may no longer be managing.

In many high-income countries, there is a recognition that older adults want to stay at home for the longest time possible. However, given the functional limitations with which they present, is ageing at home really the best place for both them and the carer? Are people wishing to stay home because the alternatives do not respond to their needs? Faced with more interesting and appropriate housing options, would policy makers benefit more from examining the joint needs of care receivers and care partners? The questions are not easy to answer but they do require that there be recognition of the wellbeing needs of the care partner.

Residential placement can be seen as the carer relinquishing care, but while the tasks and role may change, the carer may continue to provide significant levels of care. This has been described as 'care-guardianship' in the context of dementia care where the family carer's role may be considered by some to have become redundant, yet their importance as an advocate remains [26]. This role may be significant if the carer has concerns about the quality of care provided by the facility.

Various programmes have been developed to support carers through this transition. A continuous service that can provide information about residential care and how to choose a facility before admission and provided emotional support before and after the transition are recommended [27]. Good quality care can reassure the carer and enable them to spend more quality time with the person who has moved into a care facility. The approach taken by many high-income countries during the pandemic has highlighted the fact that carers are still perceived as 'visitors' rather than an integral part of the residents' lives and wellbeing.

9.7 End of Life and Palliative Care

Supporting an older person with chronic health conditions will eventually require family members to face issues surrounding end-of-life. Palliative care is a crucial part of health care incorporating relief from physical, psychological and spiritual health-related suffering due to life-threatening illness. Palliative care encompasses not only the holistic needs of the person with an illness, but also the needs of their carers.

Talking about death and dying is a taboo topic which people often find confronting and challenging. This means that older adults may reach their end of life without having their preferences expressed or documented in a process often referred to as Advance Care Planning. This can place additional stress on family carers who may be asked to make decisions about care and medical interventions and try to make these in line with the older person's preferences. Even in early stages of dementia, being able to express preferences for care in a future hypothetical scenario may be difficult. In these circumstances carers are likely to become the proxy decision-maker. Evidence shows that when carers have a poor understanding of the advanced stages of disease, the dying person is more likely to receive burdensome interventions [28].

Open discussions and planning for end of life can be helpful in enabling carers to feel in control and well prepared for the future. The needs of carers at the end of life can be similar to those in other stages of caring. This includes information about the dying process, respite care, emotional support and access to appropriate medical and support services. As described earlier, care that meets the needs of the dying person and promotes their comfort will often align with the needs of the carer. Yet there can be conflict between family carers and healthcare professionals about what is in the best interests of the dying person. Open communication between family members, the older person and their healthcare team may reduce these tensions at end of life and enable the person to have their wishes respected and their death to be comfortable. The presence of cognitive difficulties which impair communication makes these exchanges particularly difficult.

9.8 In Bereavement

After a care recipient dies, carers can experience further grief. Loss may not only relate to the loss of a significant other or loved one but may also be due to the end of the caring role. Some people may have provided support for many years and their role as a carer may have become an intrinsic part of their identity and wellbeing. The rewarding aspects of being a carer that we described earlier can end abruptly at the death of the person they cared for.

For some carers, the death of the care recipient can be a moment of relief and a renewed focus on their other roles. It may give carers hope for re-establishing interests and friendships that may have declined while providing care. It may provide relief from care tasks that can become particularly challenging during the final days and weeks of life. Carers may feel relieved if the person they cared for was suffering with their illness. Death in these circumstances may be seen as an escape from this pain.

Guilt may also become entwined in the grieving process. When the death of a care recipient was distressing or uncomfortable, the carer may feel guilty that they had not done more to advocate for their needs [29]. Guilt may also occur if the carer experiences relief at the death as they may have an expectation that they should feel deeply upset and saddened by their relative's death. To experience relief may feel like a betrayal to the memory of a loved one. As mentioned previously, the multitude of factors that affect the impact of caring come into play in their post-caring life. Were they the carers they expected to be or that their culture or social situation expected of them?

Most people process grief and loss with support from their social network of friends and family. However, those pre-existing networks of friends may have dissipated in the face of the loved one's illness. For those who have experienced a long and complex period of caring it is likely that more formal supports for grief may be needed. These may include volunteer bereavement support services, carer support groups or professional counselling. Just as there is much diversity between carers in their experience of caring, there is also a great deal of variation in the way they experience and perceive the death of the person they supported and the end of their caring role.

9.9 Summary

The caring role is dynamic with various points of transition over time which can bring rewards as well as distress and grief. The caring experience is diverse and assumptions cannot be made about how a carer will perceive their circumstances. However, for full time and primary carers, it is likely that additional support will be needed at some point during the care trajectory. Given the right opportunity, carers are often able to identify the types of support they need. Services that provide a flexible and individualised response that meets the needs of the care recipient, whether at home, or in residential care, will also often meet the needs of the carer as well, particularly in relation to respite care. There are many intervention programmes that can improve the physical, emotional and practical needs of carers, but implementing these requires dedicated services and appropriate levels of funding. It is short-sighted for health and social care systems and governments not to provide these low cost supports for carers who provide a significant contribution to society and enormous cost savings overall. Undertaking holistic assessment of both the care recipient and carers' needs is an important starting point. This includes psychological, physical, social and spiritual health needs; information about services, supports and the health conditions affecting the care recipient; financial support and flexible respite care. With the right supports through various transitions, the experience of caring can be an opportunity for personal growth and flourishing. Societies that keep a close eye on the needs of carers to older adults will be better positioned to maintain their citizens' wellbeing, and this is for both the person and the carer.

References

1. Wimo A, Gauthier S, Prince M. Global estimates of informal care. On behalf of ADI's Medical Scientific Advisory Panel and the Alzheimer's Disease International publications team. London, Alzheimer's Disease International and the Karolinska Institutet; 2018.
2. Temple JB, Dow B. The unmet support needs of carers of older Australians: prevalence and mental health. Int Psychogeriatr. 2018;30(12):1849–60.
3. Pinquart M, Sörensen S. Gender differences in caregiver stressors, social resources, and health: an updated meta-analysis. J Gerontol B Psychol Sci Soc Sci. 2006;61(1):33–45.
4. Temple J, Dow B, Kosowicz L. Carers of older Australians: unmet support needs and carer well-being. Aust J Prim Health. 2021;27(3):178–85.
5. Collins RN, Kishita N. Prevalence of depression and burden among informal care-givers of people with dementia: a meta-analysis. Ageing Soc. 2019;1:1–38.
6. Crawley S, Sampson E, Moore K, Kupeli N, West E. Grief in family carers of people living with dementia. A systematic review. Int Psychogeriatr. 2022:1–32. Online ahead of print.
7. Hopkinson MD, Reavell J, Lane DA, Mallikarjun P. Cognitive behavioral therapy for depression, anxiety, and stress in caregivers of dementia patients: a systematic review and Meta-analysis. Gerontology. 2018;59(4):e343–62.
8. Akarsu NE, Prince M, Lawrence V, Das-Munshi J. Depression in carers of people with dementia from a minority ethnic background: systematic review and meta-analysis of randomised-controlled trials of psychosocial interventions. Int J Geriatr Psychiatry. 2015;34(6):790–806.
9. Berg-Weger M, Morley JE. Editorial: Loneliness and social isolation in older adults during the COVID-19 pandemic: implications for gerontological social work. J Nutr Health Aging. 2020;24(5):456–8.
10. Schulz R, Beach SR, Czaja SJ, Martire LM, Monin JK. Family caregiving for older adults. Annu Rev Psychol. 2020;71:635–59.
11. Skufca L. AARP family caregiving survey: caregivers' reflections on changing roles. Washington, DC: AARP; 2017.
12. The Associated Press-NORC Center for Public Affairs Research. Long-term caregiving: the true sosts of caring for aging adults. Chicago: Associated Press; 2018.
13. Kaschowitz J, Brandt M. Health effects of informal caregiving across Europe: a longitudinal approach. Soc Sci Med. 2017;173:72–80.
14. Koerner SS, Kenyon DB, Shirai Y. Caregiving for elder relatives: which caregivers experience personal benefits/gains? Arch Gerontol Geriatr. 2009;48(2):238–45.
15. Semiatin AM, O'Connor MK. The relationship between self-efficacy and positive aspects of caregiving in Alzheimer's disease caregivers. Aging Ment Health. 2012;16(6):683–8.
16. Hajek A, König HH. Informal caregiving and subjective well-being: evidence of a population-based longitudinal study of older adults in Germany. J Am Med Dir Assoc. 2016;17(4):300–5.
17. Schneider U, Kleindienst J. Monetising the provision of informal long-term care by elderly people: estimates for European out-of-home caregivers based on the well-being valuation method. Health Soc Care Community. 2016;24(5):e81–91.
18. Ratcliffe J, Lester LH, Couzner L, Crotty M. An assessment of the relationship between informal caring and quality of life in older community-dwelling adults—more positives than negatives? Health Soc Care Community. 2013;21(1):35–46.
19. Garcia L, McCleary L, Drummond N. Evidence-informed approaches for managing dementia transitions: riding the waves. Elsevier: New York; 2020.

20. Twigg J, Atkin K. Carers perceived: policy and practice in informal care. Buckingham: Open University Press; 1994.
21. Vandepitte S, Van Den Noortgate N, Putman K, Verhaeghe S, Verdonck C, Annemans L. Effectiveness of respite care in supporting informal caregivers of persons with dementia: a systematic review. Int J Geriatr Psychiatry. 2016;31(12):1277–88.
22. O'Connell B, Hawkins M, Ostaszkiewicz J, Millar L. Carers' perspectives of respite care in Australia: an evaluative study. Contemp Nurse. 2012;41(1):111–9.
23. Chien LY, Chu H, Guo JL, Liao YM, Chang LI, Chen CH, Chou KR. Caregiver support groups in patients with dementia: a meta-analysis. Int J Geriatr Psychiatry. 2011;26(10):1089–98.
24. Chyr LC, Drabo EF, Fabius CD. Patterns and predictors of transitions across residential care settings and nursing homes among community-dwelling older adults in the United States. Gerontologist. 2020;60(8):1495–503.
25. Moore KJ, Dow B. Carers continuing to care after residential care placement. Int Psychogeriatr. 2015;27(6):877–80.
26. Schofield V. Careguardianship as a phase of caregiving for people with dementia [dissertation]. Wellington: Victoria University of Wellington; 1996.
27. Afram B, Verbeek H, Bleijlevens MH, Hamers JP. Needs of informal caregivers during transition from home towards institutional care in dementia: a systematic review of qualitative studies. Int Psychogeriatr. 2014;27(6):1–12.
28. van der Steen JT, Onwuteaka-Philipsen BD, Knol DL, Ribbe MW, Deliens L. Caregivers' understanding of dementia predicts patients' comfort at death: a prospective observational study. BMC Med. 2013;11:105.
29. Moore KJ, Davis S, Gola A, Harrington J, Kupeli N, Vickerstaff V, King M, Leavey G, Nazareth I, Jones L, Sampson EL. Experiences of end of life amongst family carers of people with advanced dementia: longitudinal cohort study with mixed methods. BMC Geriatr. 2017;17(1):135.

10 Conclusion to This Volume and Introduction to What Matters Volume: Population, Policy, and Systems on Care

Julie Byles

This volume has discussed healthy ageing, largely from the point of view of the individual, considering not only the length of their life but also the quality of their life, their roles and identity, and the things that make life worth living. This volume embraces the idea that what matters is "not the years in your life", but the "life in your years" [1].

Importantly, ageing is so much more than the number of candles on the cake. In 2021, the World Health Organization looked at bringing in a new code for the International Classification of Diseases (ICD-11) replacing a rarely used existing code for "senility" with a new code of "old age". This new code would recognise the contribution that the accumulation of time has on the molecular, cellular, and biological functioning of the human body, with many processes slowing down, becoming less effective or failing in later life—and so, with this purpose in mind, the code was rephrased to represent age-associated decline in intrinsic capacity [2]. The effects of these intrinsic changes are felt daily by older people who have trouble walking far, carrying out daily tasks, and putting their shoes on. They are manifest in diminished immunity, reduced cardiac and respiratory function, and cognitive decline. These impacts on intrinsic capacity undoubtedly have serious and real impact for older individuals. Potentially, scientists will eventually identify a way to slow or reverse these processes, with some promising compounds under investigation [3]. However, even when it is possible to modify the cellular effects of ageing, other factors will still matter. Healthy ageing is much more than just biology.

In longitudinal research, we see that changes in mental health and social functioning do not always track changes in physical functioning. Most people maintain high levels of mental health-related quality of life [4] and social functioning [5]

J. Byles (✉)
School of Medicine and Public Health, The University of Newcastle, Newcastle, NSW, Australia
e-mail: julie.byles@newcastle.edu.au

J. Byles (ed.), *What Matters for Healthy Ageing*, Topics in Geriatric Care,
https://doi.org/10.1007/978-981-96-0462-3_10

even in the face of low or declining physical functioning. Even people with significant age-associated limitations may still have enormous capacity for enjoyment in life. Moreover, the potential to promote and preserve mental health and social function, irrespective of physical functioning, expands the opportunities to improve the experience of ageing by orders of magnitude.

A caveat to these opportunities for healthy ageing lies in the lifelong and cumulative effects of socio-economic advantage or disadvantage, as explored in Chap. 2. For instance, there is strong evidence that socio-economic advantage in childhood is associated with better cognitive functioning in later life. Part of this association may be explained by cognitive reserve, whereby better education and intellectual stimulation may result in higher levels of cognitive capacity. This explanation is consistent with the sensitive period model discussed in Chap. 2, whereby childhood conditions have a direct effect on late life experiences. In addition, childhood socio-economic conditions affect adult conditions including highest education level, job type, and socio-economic position, consistent with the pathway model of causality. What's more, people who start in poverty and disadvantage, and who remain in these circumstances tend to accumulate risks and adversity throughout their lives, with limited opportunity to develop cognitive capacity, and multiple assaults on cognitive wellbeing. These effects are of course intergenerational, often deriving from the parents' socio-economic circumstances, and commence in utero [3]. Similar factors will apply to nutrition, bone and muscle development, respiratory and cardiovascular function, immunity, etc. (see Fig. 10.1). Genetic characteristics may also have a part to play in longevity and intrinsic capacity in older age through a complex network of interacting intracellular signalling pathways and higher order processes [6] and with gene–environment interactions also playing a role. While it is commonly cited that genes account for 25% of the difference in longevity and successful ageing, the interactions with the environment (epigenetics) amplify the impacts of both genetics and environmental factors [7].

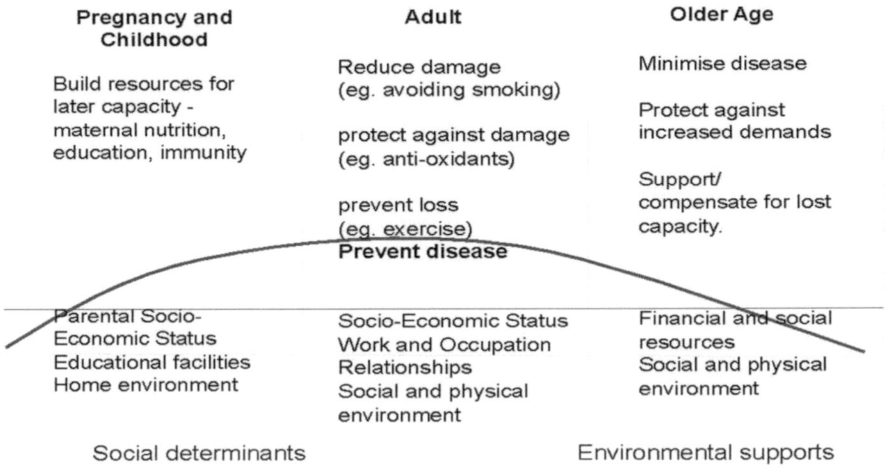

Fig. 10.1 A lifelong view of health. (Based on: Kickbusch and Kalache 1997)

Recognising the foundational, cumulative, and lifecourse influences on later life wellbeing is fundamental to understanding and enabling healthy ageing. Healthy ageing is a goal that must be strived for across ones' whole life. It is also a goal that may be more easily achieved by those who have started with and maintained advantages and harder to achieve for those who have survived through disadvantage. And yet, individuals who survive adversity may develop resilience which can help through age-related changes.

By definition older people are survivors, and most will have encountered serial stressors across their lives, finding ways to deal with events that disrupt their equilibrium. These stressors may include difficulties with work, retirement, family discord or disruption, loss of a partner, loss of ability to drive, ill health and onset of disability. According to the Salutogenic Model of Health [8], surviving these experiences helps to shape a "sense of coherence" whereby life is seen as comprehensible, manageable, and meaningful [9]. Indeed, applying a deficit model, old age can be seen as one loss after another. However, people with a strong sense of coherence, and other generalised and specific resources can find their way through [10].

For example, loss of ones' spouse is one of the most stressful of all life events. Studies of women who have lost their husbands show how women negotiate this epic change losing not only their lover and life partner, but also a major source of expressive and instrumental support. Applying the salutogenic model, Kennaugh (2016) sought to understand how older Australian women experienced ageing in the face of changing relationship status, from married to widowed. The women described the many sources of support including internal resources that helped them make sense of their lives and carry on. Friends, family and health services were important, but so were the women's abilities to learn new skills, adapt to change, and maintain a sense of optimism [11].

Another major life stressor in later life can be giving up work and transitioning to retirement. As discussed in Chap. 3, how and when people retire will be shaped not only by their individual capacities and choices, but also by the prevailing economic circumstances and job markets, and attitudes to older workers. In some cohorts, there was a policy push for people to retire early, but more recently there has been a policy focus on encouraging people to work longer. Working at older ages is seen not only as a right for older people, but also as an economic imperative for many societies. Maintaining the capacity to work, workability, is in parallel with healthy ageing, affected by both the person's intrinsic capacities, the nature of the work, and the environment in which the work is conducted. Also like healthy ageing, workability is a capacity that must be developed and preserved across the lifecourse, dependent upon education and training, health, adaptability, and limiting occupational and other assaults. As with salutogenesis, maintaining the ability to work is also dependent on motivation and the comprehension of how work fits into the person's life story and identity.

Health in older age is an important human resource, extending the individual's capacity to continue to earn and contribute. Work will, hopefully, return personal satisfaction and social connection for the individual, and benefits for the community. These advantages of work may be inhibited by ageism, including stereotyped views about when older people should stop work and their potential to contribute.

The transition to retirement is a significant life stage, which may be initiated by the older person through choice or thrust upon them through circumstances. Retirement can be a time of stress, as well as a time of growth and opportunity. Sometimes all at once. The direction and magnitude of effects of retirement on various health outcomes are likely to depend in part on the pre-retirement and concurrent circumstances, including one's pre-retirement health, work conditions and work status, as well as access to financial and social supports. In one study using data from the Sax Institute 45 and Up Study, retirement was associated with reduced odds of smoking, physical inactivity, excessive sitting, and poor sleep. More positive change in risk factors was observed for people who retired for lifestyle reasons, than those who retired for health, caring, or redundancy [12].

Chapter 5 considered the process of lifelong learning as important for healthy ageing, including enhancing older people's social connections and participation in meaningful activities. Lifelong learning is also part of salutogenesis, understanding oneself and one's life story. Not all learning has to be formal, and noting that in many societies and at different points in time, people had very limited formal education. Informal lifelong learning may be passive, including watching documentaries, reading books, listening to the radio/podcasts, or talking with others; or learning can be active through participation in hobbies, interest groups or through organisational structures such as the University of the Third Age. This lifelong learning can embrace activities that might be classed as "creative ageing", which provide an opportunity for self-expression. These activities can not only lead to joyful engagement, personal growth, and social connection, but may also help to maintain cognitive function.

The need to provide care may be a common reason for leaving paid work. Alternatively, caregiving may automatically fall to a family member who is not in paid work. In Australia, among people aged 45 to 64 years, around 8% of men and 14% of women will regularly care for a sick or disabled person. Carers will be less likely to be in the workforce compared to people without caring responsibilities, with this effect being stronger for women than for men. These full-time carers were more likely to be in poor health than similar age and sex without caring roles. The likelihood of being a carer increases with age [13]. Even in their 70s and early 80s, women are twice as likely to care for someone else than to need care themselves [14].

Caring for others is a fundamental human value, often seen as part of a loving reciprocal family relationship. As older people find it harder to undertake everyday activities due to illness or disability, their family and friends will help them with their daily activities and to maintain their dignity and quality of life. In turn, carers can find personal value and satisfaction in their caregiving role. In the Australian Longitudinal Study on Women's Health, for example, older women described caring as a central part of their lives. However, they also noted that the giving and receiving of care was reciprocal, "we care for each other". They framed their caring role within the context of long and loving relationships. Or, in some cases, the need to provide care to an ill or disabled partner, may add another level of complexity and vulnerability to what has already been a difficult relationship [14].

Caregiving is not one thing. It can be practical, helping people to shop or with transport, or with dressing and bathing, and with medical needs. It can also be emotional and social, providing people with companionship, support, and emotional strength. Caregiving also varies in terms of the intensity, duration, and demands, and according to the nature of the relationship and the caregiver's roles.

While most carers will express satisfaction with their role, their lives are still impacted by their caregiver role. Even small amounts of social support and help from formal services will go a long way to enabling carers to carry on their caregiver role. The value that carers place on their role as carers and the importance to their identity may also be important in buffering them against the demands of caregiving. The good aspects of caregiving, such as companionship and an appreciation for what they do have, may also moderate the burden and strain of caregiving.

The value of caregiving to society cannot be overestimated. In many settings, the only source of regular care for daily activities is through family and community. In Ghana, for example, older adults who experience difficulties in engaging in life activities often rely on family caregivers to fulfil their primary care needs. These needs include assistance with medication, personal care, household chores, and companionship. The carer expresses a commitment to caregiving, ensuring that the needs of older adults come first, and caregivers' personal needs come second. Consequently caring is seen as a period of transformation, and one with positive and negative impacts to some caregivers, caregiving is a medium for exposure to new skills and knowledge in life. For many caregivers, the role also means sacrificing their own social interactions, work and family roles, and creative outlets. Motivations to care include reciprocity, sense of duty, and recognition that the carer themselves will 1 day need care. However not all motivations are positive, with some fear of retribution from family members if care is not provided [14].

Chapter 4 described how social participation is of great importance for healthy ageing. Fundamental to the WHO definition is the ability for older people to continue to grow and build relationships, with these relationships being important for companionship and economic wellbeing as well as a source of support. Beyond one-to-one connections, older people also need to feel a connection to their communities, and to be perceived as a part of society with the ability to make valued contributions. Social connection can drive a virtuous cycle where health is enhanced by connections with others. Equally but oppositely, in a vicious cycle, social participation may be hindered by age-associated changes, with people finding it difficult to interact socially if they are hard of hearing, have vision or mobility difficulties, for example [15]. An essential component of healthy ageing is to break down or get around these would be barriers to enable people to participate despite their physical or cognitive difficulties.

Social interactions, support, and reciprocity can be affected by the individuals themselves, depending on their social skills and the amount of energy they put into relationships. Conditions such as depression, may impede peoples' motivation and drive to engage with others, and can also amplify feelings of loneliness and isolation [16]. Social isolation, social support, and loneliness are related but not synonymous concepts. Loneliness is perhaps the most important construct for poor quality of life [17].

Social connections can also be enhanced or impeded by the attitudes of other people and the nature of the built and social environment. Barriers may be physical, such as lack of transport, steps, or difficult paths; virtual, including being on the wrong side of the "digital divide" if older people do not have computer skills and internet access; or cultural, if older people don't feel welcomed by the prevalent images and signals, and by the behaviours of other people in public spaces.

In modern societies, connections, contributions, and identity are also related to the ability to drive or to use other forms of transport. Driving has not traditionally been seen as an expression of healthy ageing, but as presented in Chap. 6 driving is highly dependent on the persons' capacities, modified by their environment, and of great importance to their identity and social roles.

As people advance through life, memories can become increasingly important and at the front of mind. This process of remembering can be a mechanism for making sense of current circumstances within the context of a whole life. The rumination on the past may therefore be adaptive and help with resilience. As explored in Chap. 8, the revisiting of these memories may include a certain amount of rewriting to help meaning-making such that the narrative of the memories fits with the person's evolving identity and their present situation. Not all memories will be happy, but the importance is in their meaning and resonance. Not all memories will be helpful, and these more intrusive and traumatic memories may need to have a chance to be resolved.

Sexuality is an issue that is often left out of considerations of healthy ageing. Not because it isn't important to older people, but more likely because we have yet to become comfortable talking about sex as part of the human experience. When people do consider older people as sexual beings, it is often from a heteronormative frame, and often as something more in their past than their present. The considerations of sex and ageing also vary for men and women. For men, sexual dys/function is more readily recognised through the symptom of erectile dysfunction. For women, sexuality is less readily discussed except through a discourse on replacing reproductive hormones to reduce some of the biological effects of female ageing. Enhancement of sexual function may be a happy by-product.

Few researchers ask older people about sex. In one study, where men and women were asked about their interest in and opportunities for sex, 41% of men in their 80 s rated sex as currently important compared to 22% of similarly aged women. Around 20% of the men and 10% of the women had been sexually active in the past 12 months. For women, sexual activity was more likely if they were married or in a de facto relationship, but marital status did not affect the likelihood of men being sexually active [18]. A similar study using data from the English Longitudinal Study for people aged 50 years to more than 90 years found that sexual activity declined with age, and poorer health, and was less common among women compared to men. Sexually active women reported difficulties becoming sexually aroused (32%) and achieving orgasm (27%). Sexually active men reported difficulty with erectile function (39%) [18]. In both these samples, there is an assumption of heteronormative relationships, with researchers being typically reluctant to ask older people about sexual orientation or preferences. In the 45 and Up Study, when researchers included a question on sexual orientation in the first follow-up survey, most people were happy to answer. Indeed the missing data/"do not want to answer" rate (5%) for sexual orientation was far less than for income (15%) and about the same as a question on housing affordability. Around 5% of men and women described themselves as other than completely heterosexual [19].

10.1 Other Matters

Chapter 2 showed how socio-economic factors can have an effect on diet and nutrition in later life. Nutrition is of considerable importance for older people, who often have a declining appetite and a reduced ability to digest and derive nutrients from food [20]. Consequently, malnutrition is a risk for older people [21]. However, in terms of what matters, it isn't nutrition or diet, but food that is of the greatest consequence. Food is one of the most important sources of sensory enjoyment and hedonomic wellbeing, and one that can last well into later years even despite declining sense of taste. Older people may have diminished abilities or motivations to cook for themselves, especially if they live alone and have little social interaction [24]. Cooking skills may decline with loss of physical abilities or with decline in cognition [22]. Moreover, some people, such as married men, may never have developed the ability to cook for themselves. Cooking programmes can be a powerful hook to encourage older people to engage socially, learn about nutrition and other ways to look after their health, and to maintain their mental wellbeing and sense of fun [23, 24].

So as often mistakenly attributed to Marie Antionette "let them eat cake". Older age is not the time to worry about the waistline. Rather it is better to have some nutritional reserve, particularly if people have chronic disease. Numerous studies show that older people who are in the overweight range of the WHO Body Mass Index categories have longer life expectancy and healthy life expectancy. Alcohol fits into the same category as food, if a glass of wine, beer, or spirit is consistent with a person's lifestyle and culture then this practice can be extended into late life.

There may be many other topics that could expand this volume. We have not touched on sleep, bladder and bowel health, physical activity, skin integrity, and general hygiene. These factors are all important and matter for healthy ageing. Some will be considered in other volumes on morbidity, mobility, medications, and mind.

One final matter to consider is gender. Gender shapes our identity throughout life, including our attitudes (gender norms), our educational opportunities, occupations and health behaviours, and our roles (such as caregiving). As a general rule, for current cohorts, men are more likely to have higher education and greater formal workforce participation leading to a higher economic status, but men may also have worse health risk behaviours such as smoking and alcohol use. Women traditionally have fewer economic resources, including social protection, carry a greater reproductive burden, and undertake more domestic and career roles. Women are also more likely to be widowed in older age, with further loss of social status and economic resources. In addition, women generally have higher rates of disability than men throughout adulthood, and these differences may increase in later life. Paradoxically, women tend to live longer than men do.

These gender differences in ageing can have important implications for promoting health across the life course, and for meeting the specific health and care needs of older men and women. Gender mainstreaming in health can help to strengthen programme planning and implementation, reduce delay, improve diagnosis and access to services, as well as adherence and treatment outcomes. Given the influence of gender on the health of older people, action on ageing and health needs to include due attention to gender.

10.2 Considerations for Volume II

This first volume on *What Matters for Healthy Ageing* has considered matters of individual circumstance, behaviour, and identity. The next volume will move out to consider the environmental, population, system, and policy factors that also make a difference. In this volume, we recognised that older people's experience of ageing can be shaped by the attitudes of themselves and the people around them, with many of the limits to ageing well imposed by ageism rather than ageing. The built environment can also impose barriers or facilitators to physical activity, social connection, and community engagement. The environment can also be a real or perceived hazard, affecting older people's confidence and safety. The next version will also discuss systems and services that can support people in older age, and the factors to consider in ensuring they are accessible, adequate, well integrated, and effective in making a positive difference to older people's lives.

References

1. Stieglitz EJ. Preventive medicine in later maturity. Health Educ J. 1947;5(4):151–6. https://doi.org/10.1177/001789694700500403. Accessed 27 Jan 2023.
2. Rabheru K, Byles JE, Kalache A. How "old age" was withdrawn as a diagnosis from ICD-11. Lancet Healthy Longev. 2022;3(7):e457–9. https://doi.org/10.1016/S2666-7568(22)00102-7.
3. Campisi J, Kapahi P, Lithgow GJ, Melov S, Newman JC, Verdin E. From discoveries in ageing research to therapeutics for healthy ageing. Nature. 2019;571(7764):183–92. https://doi.org/10.1038/s41586-019-1365-2.
4. Leigh L, Hudson IL, Byles JE. Sleeping difficulty, disease and mortality in older women: a latent class analysis and distal survival analysis. J Sleep Res. 2015;24(6):648–57. https://doi.org/10.1111/jsr.12324.
5. Gruszczyńska E, Rzeszutek M. Trajectories of health-related quality of life and perceived social support among people living with HIV undergoing antiretroviral treatment: does gender matter? Front Psychol. 2019;10:1664. https://doi.org/10.3389/fpsyg.2019.01664.

6. Aartsen MJ, Cheval B, Sieber S, Van der Linden BW, Gabriel R, Courvoisier DS, Guessous I, Burton-Jeangros C, Blane D, Ihle A, Kliegel M, Cullati S. Advantaged socioeconomic conditions in childhood are associated with higher cognitive functioning but stronger cognitive decline in older age. Proc Natl Acad Sci U S A. 2019;116(12):5478–86.
7. Passarino G, De Rango F, Montesanto A. Human longevity: genetics or lifestyle? It takes two to tango. Immun Ageing. 2016;13:12.
8. Antonovsky A. A somewhat personal odyssey in studying the stress process. Stress Med. 1990;6(2):71–80.
9. https://doi.org/10.1007/978-3-030-79515-3_3.
10. https://link.springer.com/chapter/10.1007/978-3-030-79515-3_19.
11. Kennaugh R. "It's not how old we are; it's how we are old": a salutogenic approach to how older Australian women experi-ence ageing and respond to life stressors [doctoral thesis]. Newcastle: University of Newcastle; 2016. Australia [doctoral thesis].
12. Ding D, Grunseit AC, Chau JY, Vo K, Byles J, Bauman AE. Retirement-a transition to a healthier lifestyle?: evidence from a large australian study. Am J Prev Med. 2016;51(2):170–8.
13. Schofield D, Shrestha R, Callander E, Byles J, Kimman M. Costs of being a carer: labour force participation and lost earnings among older working-aged Australians. Aust N Z J Public Health. 2013;37(2):192–3.
14. Tooth L, Loxton D, Chan H-W, Coombe J, Dobson A, Hockey R, Townsend N, Byles J, G Mishra. From child care to elder care: findings from the Australian longitudinal study on women's health. Report prepared for the Australian Government Department of Health, May 2018.
15. Awuviry-Newton K, Tavener M, Wales K, Byles J. Using ethics of care as the theoretical lens to understand lived experiences of caregivers of older adults experiencing functional difficulties. PLoS One. 2022;17(5):e0267658.
16. Freak-Poli R, Ryan J, Tran T, Owen A, McHugh Power J, Berk M, Stocks N, Gonzalez-Chica D, Lowthian JA, Fisher J, Byles J. Social isolation, social support and loneliness as independent concepts, and their relationship with health-related quality of life among older women. Aging Ment Health. 2022;26(7):1335–44.
17. Townsend BG, Chen JT, Wuthrich VM. Barriers and facilitators to social participation in older adults: a systematic literature review. Clin Gerontol. 2021;44(4):359–80.
18. Flicker L, McCaul KA, Hyde Z, et al. Sexual activity in men and women aged 82–87 years in Western Australia. Australas J Ageing. 2010;29(2):54.
19. Lee DM, Nazroo J, O'Connor DB, Blake M, Pendleton N. Sexual health and well-being among older men and women in England: findings from the English longitudinal study of ageing. Arch Sex Behav. 2016;45(1):133–44.
20. Byles J, Forder PM, Grulich A, Prestage G. "It's okay to ask". Inclusion of sexual orientation questions is feasible in population health surveys. Aust N Z J Public Health. 2013;37(4):390–1.
21. Cristina NM, Lucia D. Nutrition and healthy aging: prevention and treatment of gastrointestinal diseases. Nutrients. 2021;13(12):4337.
22. Bardon LA, Corish CA, Lane M, Bizzaro MG, Loayza Villarroel K, Clarke M, Power LC, Gibney ER, Dominguez CP. Ageing rate of older adults affects the factors associated with, and the determinants of malnutrition in the community: a systematic review and narrative synthesis. BMC Geriatr. 2021;21(1):676.
23. Cordier R, Chen YW, Clemson L, Byles J, Mahoney N. Subjective memory complaints and difficulty performing activities of daily living among older women in Australia. Aust Occup Ther J. 2019;66(2):227–38.
24. Chojenta C, Mingay E, Gresham E, Byles J. Cooking for one or two: applying participatory action research to improve community-dwelling older adults' health and well-being. Health Promot J Austr. 2018;29(1):105–7.

MIX
Papier aus verantwortungsvollen Quellen
Paper from responsible sources
FSC® C105338

If you have any concerns about our products,
you can contact us on
ProductSafety@springernature.com

In case Publisher is established outside the EU,
the EU authorized representative is:
Springer Nature Customer Service Center GmbH
Europaplatz 3, 69115 Heidelberg, Germany

Printed by Libri Plureos GmbH
in Hamburg, Germany